Natural Progesterone for Women

YOUNG AGAIN PRODUCTS
310 N. FRONT ST. #150
WILMINGTON, NC 28401
(910) 371-2702 FAX ONLY
WWW.YOUNGAGAIN.COM
WWW.YOUNGAGAIN.ORG

NO MORE HORSE ESTROGEN!

A safe, natural and effective means of helping women with PMS, menstrual dysfunction, menopause and aging.

By

Roger Mason

NO MORE HORSE ESTROGEN!
by
Roger Mason

Copyright 2001 by Roger Mason
Young Again Products, Inc.
Wilmington, NC 28403
All Rights Reserved
Second Revision Spring 2003

No part of this book may be reproduced in any form without
the written consent of the publisher.

ISBN 1-884820-65-4
Library of Congress Control # 2001095793
Categories: 1. Health 2. Progesterone
Printed in the U.S.A.

No More Horse Estrogen! is not intended as medical
advice. It is written solely for informational and educational
purposes. Please consult a health professional should the need
for one be indicated. Because there is always some risk involved,
the author and publisher are not responsible for any adverse
affects or consequences resulting from the use of any of the
suggestions, preparations or methods described in this book. The
publisher does not advocate the use of any particular diet or
health program, but believes the information presented in this
book should be available to the public.

All listed addresses, phone numbers and fees have been
reviewed and updated during production. However the data is
subject to change.

Safe Goods Publishing
561 Shunpike Road
Sheffield, MA 01257
(413) 229-7935 or (888) NATURE-1

IV

Contents

V

Foreword

This book contains many facts and much information on progesterone and natural health for women you will not find anywhere else. In this book you'll find an easy to understand distillation of what the scientists of the world have discovered about progesterone, diet, natural hormone balance, proven supplements and how these can help you live a longer and better life in many ways.

Women have been misled and lied to long enough about the fallacies of being estrogen deficient, given horse estrogen, prescribed toxic progestin analogs, not having their hormone levels tested, not being given the other hormones they are deficient in, castrated without reason, drugged up and being told menopause is a pathological condition.

This is a short, concise book and you will not find personal stories, anecdotal evidence, entertaining stories or exciting recipes. You will find documented facts that will help you be healthier naturally without drugs or surgery. Everything you read here is backed up by published clinical studies in the international medical journals of the world. Over 90% of the current books on women's health and menopause (most of which, unfortunately, are written by women) promote "The Estrogen Myth" that women are universally deficient in estrogen, and this is what you need to be well again.

You will notice there is no profit motive in this book and no recommended sources for products or services (except for the necessary mention of the current laboratories which do saliva testing for hormones).

Please remember that bio-identical hormones, real progesterone, and natural supplements can dramatically improve your health and change your life. Holistic health, however, is based on good diet, exercise and a healthy life generally - hormones and supplements are secondary to your total lifestyle. Take personal responsibility for your health and welfare and you can change your entire destiny.

Spring 2003 revision

Topic 1: About Menopause

In 1839 a French doctor by the name of Menville coined the term "menopause". He said, "When the vital forces seek to work together in the interest of the uterus, they go to join those of the mind and the rest of the body. The critical age passed, women have the hope of a longer life than men, their thought acquires more precision, more scope and vitality." This is a pleasantly enlightened view of the natural changes every woman goes through, and contrasts very strongly with the current prevalent view generally held by Western societies today.

Menopause is merely a normal, natural, desired change in the female life cycle like puberty, yet today we celebrate puberty and dread menopause. What woman over the age of 50 would choose to bear children? This is a time for childbearing to stop (menopause is merely the cessation of menses) and a time to begin for more fulfillment, travel, self development, discovery, introspection, enjoyment, reading and leisure time....where experience, wisdom, serenity and appreciation for life can be put to use more creatively than in the younger years. Many less technologically developed cultures appreciate and respect the mature women in their society for their wisdom, judgment, humor, advice and long experience. These matriarchs are the society's honored storytellers, advice givers and sages. Maturity is obviously an asset with many advantages, not a liability with many disadvantages.

There are now almost 40 million menopausal women in America and over 30 million baby boomers very close to menopause. Now that women are living to an average age of about 78 in America this means they will spend more than one third of their lives after experiencing the end of their periods. Over one third of your life will be lived after menopause. This time can be spent very valuably, healthfully and enjoyably if you choose to. It is said that, "youth is wasted on the young", and there is a lot of truth in this. The last third of your life can be the most enjoyable period of your life and certainly not the least enjoyable.

1

Menopause in technologically developed societies is generally viewed by medical practitioners as an illness or disease - a time when hot flashes, mood swings, bone disease and cardiovascular problems predominate. This experience, however, seems to be confined to the affluent Western industrialized countries ironically enough. In poorer, less developed countries women far less commonly have such problems as they reach the age of 50. In fact it is around the age of 52 that most American women actually experience their last menstrual period, although this can literally occur in women in their thirties. This change can last a few months or as long as a few years to be complete. The months or years of change going into menopause is called pre-menopause or perimenopause, and is characterized by irregular menstruation. This is not a problem in itself. Common complaints include hot flashes, mood swings, tiredness, problematic periods, waning sexual desire and satisfaction and various other such conditions. Basically these problems are caused by estrogen dominance more than anything else. The spectrum of experience is so wide that some women experience no real problems at all going thru menopause, while others actually have to be hospitalized.

The usual medical treatment until 2003 was hormone replacement therapy with horse estrogen and artificial progestins, as well as mind numbing drugs such as Valium and Prozac. Rarely are any hormone levels tested for such basic hormones as estradiol, estrone, estriol, DHEA, testosterone, pregnenolone, melatonin or thyroid hormones. The fact doctors prescribed powerful horse estrogen and estradiol without even testing a woman's levels is criminally negligent. The supposed "benefits" of HRT have been shown to be illusory and the serious side effects not discussed. Under this treatment women just got worse and worse, and most refused to refill their prescriptions and continue with it. Most women are, in fact, excessive in estrogens and deficient in progesterone when approaching and after menopause. Natural progesterone - not artificial progestins - can be of great benefit here, especially when all the other basic hormones just mentioned are tested and balanced.

The period before menopause is called perimenopause or the climacteric. This can last up to ten years and is the gradual change to full menopause. This can start in a woman's late thirties

2

or even the late forties. Some women breeze thru this time with minimal problems, while others have endless difficulties. Irregular periods are a hallmark of perimenopause. Fatigue, occasional heavy flow, spotting, early hot flashes, emotional changes, poor sleep patterns, urinary incontinence, mood swings, dental problems, vaginal changes, variations in libido, headaches, joint pain and digestive disturbances can all be a part of this transition. Osteoporosis generally starts before the age of 40 and the symptoms finally become obvious.

As always, an ounce of prevention is worth a pound of cure. This is the time to prepare as much as possible for actual menopause. This is the time to choose better foods, start a full supplement program, get all your basic hormones balanced, monitor your hormones yearly, get off any medications, limit any bad habits, exercise regularly, start fasting one day a week and generally enjoy a total holistic lifestyle.

We can sum up the fear of menopause in three areas in Western society pretty well. Sexual attractiveness and enjoyment, decline of mental and physical health, and losing the usefulness that has put meaning in their lives. Women do identify more with their bodies than men do. As women age they feel more of a loss as they lose their physical attractiveness. Sexual desire and enjoyment do diminish as people age in all cultures. The idea that we should have as much sexual activity as we did in our twenties and enjoy it just as much is a fantasy. Sexual desire declines as we age in both men and women, and with it sexual performance and enjoyment. This is something that starts in your twenties and continues throughout life. Authors who tell you that you can have the same level of erotic activity in your mature years as you did fifty years ago are giving you an impossible ideal to live up to.

Mental and physical abilities do decline seriously in the great majority of Westerners because of their unhealthy lifestyles. Yes, there is a decline of these powers in all cultures, but not as extreme as in Western societies. In technologically developed countries older people usually are seen as "over the hill", of far less use and value and often as just old fogeys waiting to die. Retirement is a time to give up your old role in society and take on a new one. There is no better time for self development and relaxation. This is the time to enjoy your time rather than worry

3

about producing things or being of utilitarian value. It is a perfect time to give of yourself with charity and philanthropic work.

When you live in your postmenopausal years you can avoid the major problems of cardiovascular disease, breast cancer, senility, Alzheimer's, osteoporosis and other conditions. These illnesses are NOT a normal nor expected part of your mature years no matter how predominant they are in the vast majority of women.

Less than 100 years ago our forebears did not experience the current epidemic of PMS, osteoporosis, Alzheimer's, dementia, arthritis, diabetes, stroke, heart disease and other negative symptoms women experience so commonly today. This proves in itself that these conditions are certainly not normal or expected and simply do not have to happen. If they weren't common 100 years ago, why are they so common today? We have so much more knowledge of health, hygiene, nutrition, biology and other sciences that we should be much healthier than we were a century ago. It is technically true that we live longer, but our health and quality of life certainly aren't better. Length of life without quality of life just has no meaning.

One major problem with menopause and old age is the morbid fear of death most people have. The insidious, powerful fear of death and ceasing to exist predominates in Western societies to a point of obsession. No matter what people profess as to religious preference, there remains an extremely deep fear of dying. This is a time for spiritual development to deal with this irrational fear. This is the chance to realize that we are, in essence, spiritual beings beyond both birth and death. We are not merely physical bodies and temporal personalities with an average lifespan of seventy plus years. This completely irrational dread of death is cultural insanity. The older we get the more we realize we will stop existing as physical bodies and personalities. The more you identify with being a mere personality in a very temporary physical body the more you will fear death, the more you will suffer, and the more you will dread the "final ending" instead of seeing it as a TRANSITION to another level.

Topic 2: The Estrogen Myth

In 1964 a gynecologist named Robert Wilson published a book called "Feminine Forever" telling women that menopause was a disease, women were no longer feminine after menopause and that horse estrogen was the Magical Cure for these conditions. Then Ann Walsh in 1965 followed up with her book "Now! The Pills to Keep Women Young!" basically telling the same ridiculous story. Unfortunately, both of these completely undocumented and scientifically unsound books were monumental successes. The pharmaceutical corporations who profited from these internationally prescribed hormone replacement drugs were even more successful. This amazing popularity occurred with absolutely no scientific basis at all, and no proof of any of the claims. There was simply no scientific evidence that women were deficient in estrogen, that estrogen supplementation had any benefits, and especially that horse estrogen from horse urine should be used instead of real human bio-identical estrogens.

By 1975 women on ERT (estrogen replacement therapy) were getting up to 800% more uterine cancer among many, many other problems. This forced the promoters to change this therapy to HRT (hormone replacement therapy) by adding unnatural progestin analogs instead of real human progesterone. Since progesterone was unpatentable this was done purely for profit. Now even wilder and more extravagant claims were made - again with no scientific basis at all - and any side effects were denied. Of course the side effects were every bit as severe as before, only different in nature, since progestins themselves have many negative side effects. Many doctors today use the terms "progesterone" and "progestin" as if they were the same hormones!

Possibly the biggest medical fallacy going is that estrogen levels in women drop severely after menopause, and these low levels are directly responsible for all the many ills modern women suffer after the age of 50 from depression to hot flashes. Countless clinical tests prove quite the opposite. The fallacy continues that horse estrogen is the Magic Answer and you don't even have to test women for their estrogen levels. The truth of the matter is that Western women in America and Europe generally have excessive estrogen levels (even after menopause) as proven by endless studies of actual blood levels - especially of estradiol and estrone. Have you noticed how very few women refilled their estrogen prescriptions? HRT "therapy" did not fulfill the many promises made, and the side effects were simply intolerable. How many women have ever told you how wonderful estrogen supplementation was, how much it helped them and how you should try it, too? The fact is the HRT was a dismal failure year after year, yet doctors continued to relentlessly prescribe it, and women continued to mindlessly take it. Finally in 2002 it was officially admitted to be a failure. Progesterone is what falls severely after menopause since the ovaries are no longer active. The solution clearly is to use real natural progesterone in normal physiological amounts and to measure levels of all three basic estrogens in case there is a deficiency in any of them. Balancing the other basic hormones is just as vital to this program.

Menopause is anything but a disease caused by low estrogen levels and cured by estrogen supplementation, especially with foreign horse estrogen like equilin the human body cannot even recognize. Medical doctors almost never test women for estradiol or estrone and certainly not for estriol, DHEA, testosterone, androstenedione, FSH, LH, cortisol, progesterone, melatonin, pregnenolone, thyroid hormones or growth hormone. The many medical studies that have been done on women after menopause show that the levels of estrone and estradiol do fall significantly, but just enough to prevent menstruation and fertilization. After menopause estrogen levels are intentionally high enough for all the other natural and needed bodily functions. Nature understandably does not want women having children at this age. We can see the natural order stops childbearing completely about the age of 50 and menopause is an important and necessary part of the natural order of life. The postmenopausal levels of estrogens are sufficient for normal functioning of your body, and it is unusual to find a deficiency that needs to be supplemented. Doctors would do immeasurable good for women by testing the levels of ALL their basic hormones and balancing them as much as possible. Fortunately, you don't need to go to an endocrinologist or even your family doctor to do so. Now you can accurately and scientifically test your own hormone levels with inexpensive saliva test kits without a prescription.

Doctors show almost no interest at all in such basic diagnosis and treatment of the whole body. What could be more central to your health than your basic hormone metabolism? Hormones affect everything in your body and your mind.

This myth of estrogen deficiency and the supposed wonders of estrogen supplementation were so deeply ingrained in the medical profession and the public mentality that it was never even questioned. The propaganda never seemed to stop. Finally in 2002 the medical profession was forced to admit that HRT was too dangerous to use anymore - after 40 years of ruining women's lives with these poisons. You no longer see the ads on TV and in magazines endlessly promoting the virtues of HRT.

Medical studies of women in poorer agrarian countries that do not experience the high rates of osteoporosis, heart disease, arthritis, hot flashes and other problems show that they have no higher estrogen levels than American and European women. This is proof that estrogen isn't the problem at all. If low estrogen was the problem, obviously these Third World women would clearly have definitely higher levels. Actually they have been shown to have equal or even lower levels. Western women, in fact, have higher estrogen levels from eating so much saturated fat, drinking alcohol, being overweight, eating too many calories, and not exercising among other factors. Excess estrogen and deficient progesterone and other hormones are a basic cause of our frightening rates of cancer, especially breast, uterine, ovarian and cervical cancers, as well as many other diseases and conditions. The much touted "benefits" of HRT simply aren't true and clinical studies show this. Finally, in 2002 the medical profession admitted as much.

You were told endlessly that estrogen supplementation prevents osteoporosis. You'll see in the chapter "Osteoporosis" that this isn't true at all, since estrogen controls osteoclasts (which merely remove dead bone cells) and not osteoblasts (which actually build new bone cells). You were also told that estrogen replacement therapy is good for heart and artery health. This is not true either, since women with heart disease can't even take estrogen supplements and heart disease is an admitted side effect. You were told that estrogen replacement therapy prevents Alzheimer's and makes you live longer. Again the facts show the opposite. The truth is that excessive estrogen levels cause breast, uterine, ovarian and cervical cancers, arthritis, obesity and a host of other ills. Various "studies" funded by the pharmaceutical companies purported to show the many benefits of HRT therapy. The unfounded studies showed a very different picture however.

Any doctor who does not test your estradiol, estrone and estriol levels yet wants to blindly prescribe estrogen or any other hormone (when your levels may already be too high) is telling you he doesn't know what he's doing nor does he care. Your doctor probably doesn't have the word "estriol" in his vocabulary. You may find a doctor who knows how to test all your basic hormone levels, or just test them yourself with saliva. If you have a low level of either estradiol, estrone or estriol as proven by a blood or saliva test, then you certainly should raise that one hormone with a human equivalent supplement. You can buy soy derived estradiol and estrone and get estriol from a compounding pharmacy (regular pharmacies do not stock estriol). Please read the chapter on "Home Hormone Testing" to see how easy this is to do yourself without a doctor. Women with hysterectomies need special attention here for all their hormones and this is covered in Topic 19: Don't Get A Hysterectomy.

You were never told of the side effects of estrogen supplementation, but these, by law, must be stated in the prescription package. Unfortunately, very few women ever bothered to read them. These inserts clearly warn of uterine cancer, breast cancer, gall bladder disease, abnormal blood clotting, heart disease and excess blood calcium as some of the known effects. In addition to these are a long, long list of other problems including nausea, skin yellowing, breast enlargement, enlargement of uterine tumors, breakthrough bleeding, abnormal cervical secretions, yeast infections, fluid retention, various skin problems, migraine headache, mental depression, muscle spasms, hair loss, blood sugar irregularities and loss of sex drive among others. Did your doctor bother to mention these to you? Did the article you read on the "wonders of HRT" list these side effects? Did the book you read on why to take HRT warn you of these problems? Or did that actress on TV mention them?

8

Topic 3: What is Estrogen?

There is no such thing as "estrogen" per se; it is just a convenient term to use for collectively talking about the total estrogen group. There are literally dozens of estrogenic hormones, but there are only three primary human estrogens we need to be concerned with and discuss.

ESTRIOL (E3), the "forgotten estrogen", comprises approximately 80 to 90% of human estrogen and is the most abundant, the safest, the weakest biologically, and can be the most beneficial. Amazingly enough, almost no doctor or pharmacist seems to even be aware that it even exists, although it is the most prominent estrogen in our bodies. What little research has been done shows just how important this is for proper female metabolism. Estriol is not even manufactured in the U.S., sold in regular pharmacies, or listed in their source books. You must find a sympathetic and open minded doctor, a compounding pharmacy to fill your prescription, and use a topical or intravaginal gel or cream. NEVER take oral estriol in any form as it is just not absorbable and is broken down into unwanted metabolites. Fortunately you can easily saliva test your levels to see that they are sufficient, or a doctor can order a blood test done when he tests your other hormone levels. Time of day and time of the month are vital here as levels vary greatly. One suggestion is if your levels are low, have 100 grams of a 0.3% transdermal (never the unnatural and dangerous oral forms) cream made and use a half gram of this daily (1.5 mg daily) for about seven months. Retest yourself after about three months to see how you're doing. We should see more research done on this in the future. One day an American company will produce an estriol cream, doctors will become aware of its importance, and this will finally become a regularly available natural hormone.

At the Fujita Health University in Japan (Nippon Naibun. Gak. Zas. vol. 72, 1996) doctors studied obese women and found literally all of them were low in estriol. Many of them were anovulatory (not producing an egg during their cycle) and therefore not producing any progesterone as well. This does not

9

mean that estriol is a magical cure for obesity, but rather that estriol is the "forgotten" estrogen and is basic to your health.

Doctors worldwide never test for estriol levels in women much less write prescriptions for it. Neither chain nor independent pharmacies stock it, nor can even special order a transdermal estriol gel or cream. You must find a doctor interested in natural hormones and explain you want a 100gram tube of 0.3% (three tenths of one per cent) transdermal natural estriol - never oral estriol salts or injections. A compounding pharmacist can make this up for you inexpensively. Do not buy useless "homeopathic" estriol creams that contain no actual hormones. Use a half gram a day intravaginally and 100 grams will last you about seven months. You can also use this on thin skin just like progesterone. It is important to retest and monitor your levels. Never use this unless your blood or saliva tests prove you are low.

ESTRONE (E1) only comprises about 5 to 10% of human estrogen and is much stronger than estriol, but weaker in effect than estradiol. Bio-identical estrone is readily available. Countless clinical studies show that American women generally have excessive levels of estrone from such factors as high fat diets. Overweight women (and a third of American women are overweight) often have excessive levels of this resulting in estrogen dominance. It is uncommon to find a deficiency, except sometimes in women with hysterectomies. Excessive levels can be reduced by making better food choices, taking saturated FAT out of your diet, losing weight, not drinking alcohol, eating lower calorie foods, and taking supplements like DIM and flax oil (see the "Natural Supplements" chapter). The most important thing is to eat a natural and healthful diet low in fats especially animal fats. The prevailing medical fallacy is that women are somehow "deficient" in estrone generally and need to be given supple-ments. The fact is that women in Western countries generally have excessive levels and need to lower them, not raise them. Do not use the dangerous anti-aromatase drugs to lower your estrogen, however, due to their toxic side effects. You can test your estrone levels just like you test for your estriol levels.

ESTRADIOL (E2) also comprises about 5 to 10% of human estrogen. This is the most powerful and most dangerous one, as it is twelve times more potent than estrone and a full

10

eighty times more potent that estriol. It is often high in women for the same reasons as estrone is and can be lowered in the same ways. Again, women are told by their physicians that they are deficient in estradiol generally and need supplementation (without even testing them) when, in fact, they usually need to lower their levels - especially of estradiol - since it is the most potent and dangerous estrogen and very carcinogenic in excess.

Horse estrogen was the most prescribed drug for women in the world with 45 million prescriptions a year until 2002 when it was finally admitted this was a dismal failure all along. Horse estrogen is actually extracted from the urine of pregnant mares. Unbelievable! Horse estrogen is composed of about half estrone and estradiol and half equilin and other equine (horse) estrogens. When you consider that a foreign animal estrogen like equilin was being given to women without even testing their levels or using real human equivalent estradiol, or balancing this with natural progesterone, it frightens you. The prescription insert admits that breast and uterine cancer are side effects as are gall bladder disease, abnormal blood clotting and heart disease. Seventeen specific side effects are also listed.

The main estrogen used in birth control pills is ethinyl estrogen and is very dangerous even at low doses. This is a completely synthetic estrogen that does not exist in nature. It is actually more potent than estradiol (E2). Find another means of contraception and do not use The Pill to avoid pregnancy. The long term use results in severe side effects including various forms of cancer.

Every author on natural health is telling you that soy isoflavones are "phytoestrogens" or plant estrogens that bind to the estrogen receptors in our bodies. Ladies, this is the biggest crock since the "earth is flat" theory. Soy isoflavones are plant pigments unrelated to hormones in any way, shape or form. Plant pigments have nothing at all to do with estrogen or any other hormone chemically or biologically. Yes, isoflavones are a valuable and proven supplement to take, but they have nothing at all to do with hormone levels, hormone receptors or anything else related to hormones. Even scientists and medical journals repeat this fallacy. This is the only book in the world to tell you the truth that there are no "phytoestrogens", never have been and never

11

will be. A similar fallacy is promoted with "xenoestrogens" which are supposed to be environmental toxins that mimic estrogen and attach to your estrogen receptors. Certainly there are many environmental toxins we have to deal with but none of them have anything at all to do with estrogen or any other hormone. Hormones are secreted by mammals and not by plants or plastic factories.

SERMs should be mentioned in this chapter. SERMs are selective estrogen receptor modulators, which are also called "designer estrogens". These are just more toxic, synthetic, unnatural prescription poisons that will make your health and life worse. These dangerous drugs turn on some of the estrogen receptors in your body and turn off others. The mechanism of their action is really not understood well at all as it is very complex. Obviously SERMs are anything but natural, and the effects they have on your body are very unbalancing. These may turn out to be even worse than horse estrogen and progestins in the end. Do not use these under any circumstances.

Don't just blame doctors, because if women would demand all their estrogen levels be tested they would never get any pre-scriptions they didn't need. Doctors would also learn about estriol, "the forgotten estrogen", and routinely test for it, prescribe it when needed, and pharmacies would carry it. There would only be human equivalent hormones and horse estrogen would no longer be sold at all. Doctors would test and balance all your basic hormones as they all work together in concert and not individually. There is a very small minority of doctors who do understand these things, and will help you if you take the time to find them. The fact that doctors routinely prescribe horse estrogen, estrone and estradiol without ever testing the women they give these to is criminal. The fact they seem completely unfamiliar with such basic hormones as DHEA, testosterone, pregnenolone, growth hormone and melatonin is equally so. Hormones are very powerful, and estrogens are dangerous in excess. You must test your levels of estradiol and estrone especially to know what they are. Usually you will find these levels are excessive even after menopause and certainly it is unusual to find deficient levels.

Topic 4: What Is Natural Progesterone?

We should always understand that whenever we use hormone supplements we should use the natural, bio-identical forms in such doses as to maintain our normal youthful levels as long as we live. This is one main pillar of life extension. Also, we need to understand that nearly all of the supplements and hormones we buy are, in fact, synthesized, but are equivalent to the natural human molecule chemically and biologically.

Synthetic vitamin C, for example, is very inexpensive and always used in supplements regardless of what you've been told by the vitamin companies. Natural vitamin C extracted from fruit, on the other hand, is a laboratory curiousity that is far too expensive to use. Progesterone cannot be extracted from cadavers, and must be synthesized from soy sterols or yam diosgenin. It is biologically identical to human progesterone.

Unfortunately, unscrupulous supplement promoters have put plain yam extract into creams and told women this is a "biological precursor" to real progesterone and the body will "convert" it. This is known as "yam scam" in the trade. Read the label on the jar, and if it says "yam", "wild yam" or any other kind of yam on the label avoid it completely. The product must clearly state exactly how many milligrams of USP natural progesterone are contained inside or don't buy it. Many creams simply refuse to state this, so you'll never really know if they are real or not. Again, the label must clearly state how much USP natural progesterone is contained in the jar and no mention of the word "yam" should appear anywhere. A good cream should state that a two ounce jar contains about 800 to 1,000 milligrams (400 to 500 milligrams per ounce in other words) and retail for less than $20 (since a gram [1,000 milligrams] of micronized progesterone only costs about forty cents wholesale).

Progesterone is not absorbed when taken orally as the liver breaks it down into unwanted byproducts, and very little progesterone is actually absorbed. Some manufacturers have tried to get around this by offering large oral doses or sublingual (under the tongue) preparations, but this just doesn't solve the problem. Injections are totally unnecessary here and very impractical. A nasal spray would have to be approved by the FDA unfortunately, as it would be considered a new drug form and require government approval (bureaucrats improving your life as usual) as well as a prescription. Vaginal and anal suppositories are completely unnecessary, and many women would not like using them. Fortunately progesterone readily penetrates the skin and enters into the bloodstream bypassing the liver. Transdermal creams are far and away the most effective, proven, safest, least expensive and most convenient way to use this.

Using a good brand of cream during days 12 to 26 of your cycle (day 1 is the first day of your actual period) follows the natural cyclical pattern you experience, since this is when progesterone is released by the ovarian follicles. A half teaspoon a day applied to thin, soft skin will give you about 30 milligrams on these 14 days, and about 20 to 25 milligrams will actually enter your bloodstream bypassing the liver. During perimenopause when periods are irregular this can become more difficult to do. After menopause you can use a quarter teaspoon any three weeks of the calendar month as an easy to follow pattern.

It is crucial to use natural hormones in natural ways in normal physiological amounts to maintain youthful levels as much as possible to stay in the best of health and to live as long as possible. Progesterone is very safe and nontoxic especially in the amounts we've talked about. There are many benefits of progesterone supplementation for most women and more benefits are being discovered for it. There are quite a number of studies proving that transdermal progesterone creams are effectively absorbed into the blood and have the dramatic effects we have been talking about. More studies are being done all the time that show that natural progesterone can be of great benefit to women including ways we haven't yet discovered.

Topic 5: What Are Progestins?

Progestins are NOT "synthetic progesterone" at all. We've seen that all bio-identical human equivalent hormones such as natural progesterone must be made in laboratories. Progestins, however, are unnatural analogs (completely different molecules) of real progesterone with the only advantage being they are orally absorbable. Progestins are very, very different chemically and biologically. They have almost none of the wonderful benefits of progesterone and have many serious side effects. Surprisingly, you will often hear medical doctors and other health professionals call progestins "progesterone". This can be inexcusable ignorance more than purposeful untruthfulness. If it is in a pill or capsule you can be sure it is not real progesterone.

Progestins do not exist anywhere in nature and were designed by scientists. Their only relationship is that their basic chemical structure is based on the progesterone molecule. The most heavily marketed of progestin is Provera, which is medroxy progesterone. You can see how very different it is in the following diagrams. Natural progesterone cannot, of course, be patented for profit, but Provera is the most widely sold patented progestin.

Natural progesterone in normal doses has no known side effects or contraindications, but any of the progestins have many such negative effects. By law these must be listed in the package insert and you will see listed five specific side effects, eight contraindications, ten adverse reactions and five consequences... That's 28 different and compelling reasons not to take them.

Liver malignancy, cystitis, depression, fatigue, headache, nervousness, dizziness, insomnia, epilepsy, asthma, cardio-pulmonary aggravation, as well as lowering the levels of real progesterone are just a few of the reasons not to take them. Add to this list fluid retention (edema), possibility of birth defects, breast cancer, blood clots, menstrual irregularities, skin problems, hair loss and weight gain and you wonder why anyone in their right mind would even consider taking a drug this dangerous - or why anyone in their right mind would prescribe it to them.

15

Obviously there is only one reason that toxic drugs like progestins are so heavily marketed and sold to unsuspecting, naïve people - instead of inexpensive, natural, bio-identical, non-prescription progesterone - and that is PROFIT. There is no other reason to give women expensive, dangerous, unnatural pre-scription analogs with a long list of side effects.

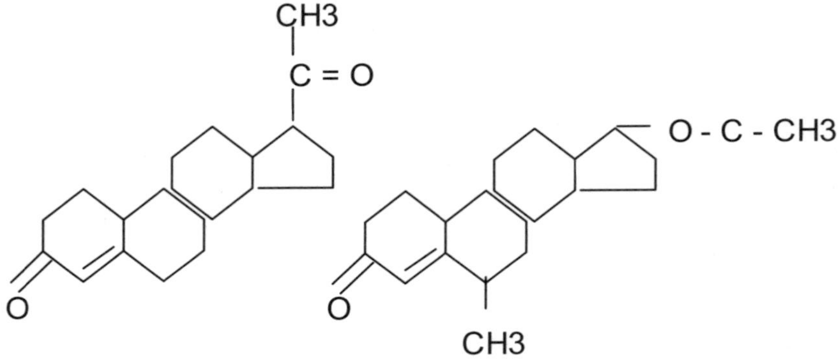

PROGESTERONE   PROVERA

The molecular structures above may seem somewhat similar to the layperson, but they are completely different. Slight changes in a chemical molecule cause extreme changes in their effects. Natural progesterone is identical to what is in our bodies even though it must be made in a laboratory - the molecule is exactly the same. Progestins are foreign molecules that have many serious side effects and are unrelated chemically to real human progesterone. The only "advantage" to progestins is that they are orally absorbable. Natural progesterone cannot be taken in a pill or tablet and should be used in a transdermal cream as the most practical means of application. There is just no choice between taking a natural hormone with many proven health benefits or a toxic, artificial poison with serious side effects. The fact that almost no medical doctors are aware of such an obvious situation should be a clear warning to you.

16

Topic 6: Estrogen Versus Progesterone

ESTROGEN	PROGESTERONE
stimulates endometrial growth	limits endometrial growth
stimulates breast growth	matures breast cells
raises blood pressure	normalizes blood pressure
retains fluid in body	diuretic
stimulates blood clotting	normalizes clotting
raises blood pressure	normalizes blood pressure
unbalances zinc/copper ratio	helps normalize ratio
stimulates uterine cancer	resists uterine cancer
stimulates ovarian cancer	resists ovarian cancer
weakens immunity	strengthens immunity
stimulates osteoclasts (removes dead bone cells)	stimulates osteoblasts (builds bone cells)
promotes tumor growth	resists tumor growth
promotes cyst growth	resists cyst growth
doesn't protect lungs	protects lung function
worsens PMS	soothes PMS
increases inflammation	cools inflammation

unbalances menses	normalizes menses
worsens arthritis	anti-inflammatory
increases menopausal symptoms	relieves menopausal symptoms
accelerates aging	slows aging process
weakens fertility	promotes fertility
promotes abortion	promotes conception
stimulates prostate disease in men	protects prostate from disease in men
correlates with obesity	correlates with normal weight

It is obvious that estrogen in excess has very toxic effects on us, while progesterone has safe and protective effects. Estrogens certainly are important for our health in moderation but are very dangerous when the levels are high or there is not enough progesterone to balance them.

Topic 7: Osteoporosis

Osteoporosis is an unnecessary, but currently epidemic, affliction in the Western world. This is not true in many other parts of the world however, especially in Third World countries like in Africa, Asia and South America. This proves bone disease is caused by factors we can and should control. Isn't it ironic that poor people in Third World countries suffer less bone and joint disease than in the developed countries? Osteoporosis, like any other illness, is not some mysterious "accident" we don't understand. Taking prescription drugs for this is not the answer at all, and NONE of them work or have ever worked. You'll find that no matter what you hear in the media about the osteoporosis drug of the year it not only won't help you, but it sure will make you worse in the end. The advertising is as persuasive as it is misleading so please don't be persuaded by it. Every year a new "miracle drug" for building bone is trotted out with much fanfare, which never lives up to any of the promises made for it. When are people going to catch on that prescription drugs do not build bone and will not build bone now or in the future? For years bisphosphonates have been promoted by doctors even though they are proven to be toxic and don't work. Salmon calcitonin has also failed. In 2003 zoledronic acid is the new Wonder Drug and will fail just as badly.

This is certainly not due to calcium deficiency as is popularly believed. Women in Western countries have the highest calcium intake of anyone on earth and the highest consumption of dairy products. These same women also have the highest rates of osteoporosis, hip fractures, bone disease and arthritis. Half of all Caucasian women over the age of 50 already have serious bone loss, as this starts at about the age of 35 on the average. This simply was not common in America 100 years ago and many factors contribute to this - most of all our current American diet.

The other prevailing myth is that osteoporosis is due to estrogen deficiency, and taking estrogen supplements, especially horse estrogen, will strengthen your bones. This is not true despite the constant propaganda you hear otherwise. For example, a 1995 study in the New England Journal of Medicine studied 9,500 women over a period of eight years and found no benefit at all for women who were taking estrogen supplements especially with regard to hip fractures. Hip fractures are the single most important injury due to osteoporosis and half of the women who suffer from them never walk again. Estrogen does not help or cure osteoporosis at all as estrogen controls the cells that remove the dead bone (osteoclasts) while progesterone stimulates the bone cells (osteoblasts) to build new bone.

The facts are that bone loss starts in most American women in their mid thirties when they have very youthful estrogen levels. Bone loss often occurs when progesterone levels are low which can be due to anovulation. Unfortunately women cannot tell if they have not ovulated. Progesterone supplementation should start therefore in most women at least by the age of forty. Starting years before menopause occurs is necessary, since this is when the bone loss is really beginning, but not yet showing any outward symptoms. As a general rule bone loss occurs at a rate of about 1.5% lost bone cells every year until women at eighty only have about HALF the bone mass they had at the age of forty! Imagine having half your bone strength. This is frightening to know you can only expect to have fifty per cent of your bone cells at that age. You can avoid this situation however by good diet and lifestyle, resistance exercise, proper supplements and hormone balancing.

We think of bones as rigid and dead rather like the anatomical skeletons we see in laboratories, but quite the opposite is true. Our bones are very alive and well; they are dynamic and constantly replace old cells with new ones. About every three months we have completely new small (trabecular) bones and about every twelve years we have completely new long (cortical) bones. We are always growing new bones.

Osteoclasts take out the old bone cells to make room for the new ones and these are controlled by estrogen. This proves estrogen cannot build new bone cells as you have been repeatedly told. Osteoblasts build new bone cells and these are controlled by progesterone. If you are low in progesterone your bone building metabolism will be limited. You can actually reverse osteoporosis in most cases and start rebuilding lost bone cells when you follow a program of healthy diet (please read my Zen

Macrobiotics for Americans), proven supplem
mone balance, avoiding bad habits, and res'
stress your bones. It is total lifestyle that w
strong all your life.

Do not think that progesterone alone
a holistic program of bone health because it is u...,
Testosterone, androstenedione, DHEA and estriol are
powerful bone building hormones. Diet is the most important
factor. It is important to reduce animal fat and protein as well as
sugar and sweets as these acidify the body and upset the normal
alkaline balance. Dairy products should be avoided no matter how
low-fat or non-fat due to the lactose content as well as the animal
proteins. Again, American and European women who eat the most
dairy products have the highest rates of osteoporosis, arthritis,
and bone disease. See www.notmilk.com or www.milksucks.com
on the Internet to see more reasons not to drink milk or eat dairy
products.

You can take 600 to 800 mg of any calcium supplement
you like, but take 300 to 400 mg of magnesium with this and 3 mg
of boron to see that the calcium is absorbed as magnesium and
boron are necessary for bio-availability. 400 to 800 IU of vitamin D
is also important. You should take all the thirteen minerals you
need including zinc, chromium, selenium, vanadium, copper,
manganese molybdenum, iron, iodine and silicon as they all work
together as a group. Strontium has value, but it will be hard to find
until the public becomes more aware of it as a supplement.
Ipriflavone is a fine supplement for bone health and is simply a
modified isoflavone. Vitamin B-6 is good but the 50 mg doses
usually recommended are simply irresponsible as they are
megadoses. 10 mg is very sufficient as this is 500% of your RDA.
Vitamin B-12 1000 mcg (as it is so poorly absorbed) or 5 mg of
methyl cobalamin is good as well and folic acid 800 mg. These
three B vitamins will also help lower your homocysteine levels and
improve your cardiovascular health. Vitamin C is good but no
more than 250 mg as any more than that will acidify your blood.
Do NOT take megadoses of vitamin C no matter what you've
read! Vitamin E 400 IU (mixed tocopherols) is valuable here as
well. Vitamin K 80-160 mcg has been shown to be important in
bone metabolism. All of the foregoing have extensive published
evidence of their importance in good bone metabolism.

.y resistance exercise will strengthen bones. One reason
in poorer countries have stronger bones is that they
y do a lot of manual labor and physical exercise just to
ive. Swimming is good and any exercise that puts weight on
ur bones and stresses them makes them stronger. Weight
.raining for women with lighter weights is the ideal exercise here
and you can join a gym or put exercise equipment in your house.
This is a most important factor in having strong bones as
American women rarely stress their bones with any resistance
exercise.

Osteoporosis and bone loss are increased by such things
as high protein intake (we eat twice the protein we need), lack of
exercise, drinking sodas (phosphoric acid, sugar and caffeine),
smoking, hysterectomies, drinking alcohol and coffee (even
decaf), high sugar intake (any sweeteners including honey),
stress, excessive salt intake, eating saturated fats, and being
overweight. This includes over 99% of American women right
there. The only way to maintain and build bone mass is by a
program of total lifestyle including good diet, proven supplements
and resistance exercise. Nothing less is going to work.

You can find out the state of your bone loss by getting
them measured by a physician. Dual photon absorptiometry (DPA)
is considered 97% accurate and uses photons (light energy) to
measure bone loss and may be preferable to using DEXA. Dual
Energy X-Ray Absorptiometry uses low level X-radiation and is
also considered to be 97% accurate.

There are dozens of published studies demonstrating that
progesterone - not estrone or estradiol - is the primary bone
building hormone. The classic study was "Progesterone as a
Bone-Tropic Hormone" from the University of British Columbia.
Similar studies have been done all over the world at top
institutions such as the University of Illinois, Clermont-Theix INRA
in France, Utrecht University Hospital in the Netherlands,
University of Utah, University of Toronto, Pennsylvania State
University, Stanford University, Tongji Medical University in Japan,
the Ernst Schering Research Foundation and the University of
Parma in Italy. The evidence is simply overwhelming here.

Topic 8: Cholesterol and Heart Health

What is the leading cause of death by far for American women? Coronary heart disease far and away. All types of heart and artery disease kill women every year more than anything else. What can you do about it? Follow the suggestions in this book and make better food choices, take proven supplements, avoid prescription medications, don't have bad habits, balance your hormones and get regular exercise that stresses your bones. That is what you can do. More specifically what can you do for better heart health? Lower your cholesterol and triglycerides - THE most important of all factors. The average cholesterol level for adult Americans runs about 225-250 mg/dl, while in many Asian countries it is more commonly about 150. Do not accept the regularly advocated figure of 200 mg/dl, as 150 is the practical ideal. What's the difference? FAT INTAKE! The 42% mostly saturated animal fats we eat is what causes such high cholesterol levels and resultant coronary heart disease. Stop eating all the red meat, poultry, eggs, milk and various dairy products. The worst fats of all are the hydrogenated or "trans fatty acids" which do not exist in nature. Real vegetarians and people who eat seafood basically have no cholesterol problems. Remember there isn't a drop of cholesterol in any plant, and it only is found in animal foods. The cholesterol in fish and seafood does not raise your levels when eaten moderately.

What about supplements that will lower cholesterol and greatly reduce the risk of heart disease? We are going to talk about five cornerstone supplements that will do this with no change in diet or exercise. If you are also willing to make changes in your diet and exercise the results are truly astounding. Anyone who takes dangerous prescription drugs for high cholesterol is making a very unnecessary and very unwise choice. These drugs are not that effective, are very expensive and have such severe side effects your liver enzymes must be monitored. It is very easy to lower your cholesterol and triglyceride levels naturally without dangerous, toxic drugs. These five supplements will also help your health in many other ways and some have already been discussed in the supplement chapter.

The first one is beta-sitosterol. If you can't find this at your health food store or vitamin catalog search the Internet for a brand with 300 mg of mixed sterols. This is simply an extract of sugar cane or soybeans that has been known about for 30 years for its powerful and beneficial effects on blood lipids (fats) from dozens of international studies. Do not use the margarines and salad dressings with added sterols as these are weak, expensive and full of fats. There is one well promoted product that only contains a useless 30 mg of beta-sitosterol, so read the label and make sure EACH tablet contains 300 milligrams of mixed beta-sitosterols.

The second proven supplement is called "guggul" gum and it is the resin from the Indian Commiphora tree. This has literally been known about in Ayurvedic medicine for two thousand years yet we are just learning about it and studying the effects clinically. You need 250 mg with 10% sterones (i.e. 25 mg of actual guggul sterones) to be effective. You can find this in any health food store and most vitamin catalogs or on the Internet. Do not take this for more than a year as it is "exogenous" and the effects wear off.

The third is flax seed oil and has already been mentioned in the supplement chapter. Buy this refrigerated and keep it refrigerated and take one or two 1,000 mg capsules a day. Two capsules will add an insignificant 18 fat calories to your diet. This is the best source of omega-3 fatty acids known, and is a much better choice than fish liver oils for a variety of reasons. Our diets have an overabundance of omega-6 fatty acids (linoleic) and a scarcity of omega-3 fatty acids (linolenic). There are many studies of the varied health benefits of flax oil supplements for our health in general aside from improved blood lipid levels.

The fourth is beta glucan and has also been mentioned in the supplement chapter. Please read my book "What Is Beta Glucan?" (Safe Goods Publishing) to learn more about the great benefits of this supplement. Besides being the most powerful immune enhancer known to science, it also does wonders for your cholesterol levels. Take 200 mg a day of either oat or yeast beta glucan as both sources are equal in power regardless of the advertising. Technology has advanced only in the last few years to extract this economically and make it available to the public as a supplement. The research on its health benefits only goes back about 15 years, so this is quite a new discovery. This is even being studied for its potent anti-cancer properties among other benefits.

The last is soy isoflavones, which were mentioned in the supplement chapter as well. Just take 40 mg a day of mixed isoflavones containing both genestein and daidzein. You are just not going to be able to eat enough soy foods to get this much unless you drink a cup of soymilk a day. One cup will add a whopping 3,600 calories a month to your diet as it contains about 120 calories or more depending on the brand. Every time you study a disease you'll usually find that soy isoflavones come up in the literature with studies showing the benefits of using them. Again, these "flavones" or plant pigments are unrelated in any way to estrogen in any form and cannot attach to estrogen receptors (see Topic 3: What Is Estrogen?).

When you look in the drug store, health food store or vitamin catalogs you will notice a very poor and very limited selection of cholesterol supplements. The few you see can be very misleading in the amounts of active ingredients they contain as well as their purported effectiveness.

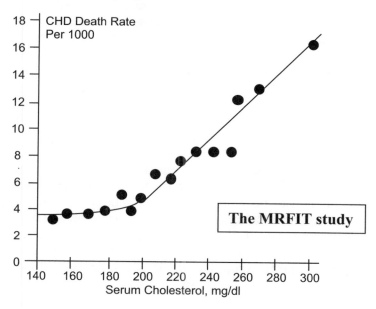

You can see very clearly by this chart from the MRFIT study that the ideal cholesterol level is about 150 mg/dl. Anything over this level results in a higher death rate from coronary heart disease, so a level of 200 is not good enough at all.

What other supplements are useful here besides these five "cornerstone" ones? Acidophilus is very important to keep our intestinal flora in balance. It is in our large intestine that fats are digested. Use a good brand with at least three billion units and keep it refrigerated. Along with the acidophilus use 750 mg of "FOS" or fructo-oligosaccharides. This is also known as inulin and is an indigestible natural sugar that feeds the good intestinal bacteria while starving the bad ones. The use of the amino acid L-glutamine is the third way to keep healthy intestines that will properly digest fats without raising our cholesterol levels. This will also spike your growth hormone levels. Take a gram of L-glutamine in the A.M. and a second gram in the P.M.

Beta carotene is a good supplement for regulating cholesterol in 10,000 IU to 25,000 IU amounts. Vitamin C is also good but no more than 250 mg a day. Vitamin E is important here and you can use 200 IU to 400 IU of mixed tocopherols for good results. Lecithin from soybeans is an old standard and you can take 1,200 mg softgels. Lecithin is also known as phosphatidyl choline. Fruit pectin from either apples or citrus fruits is good, but you must take at least three to five grams a day for effectiveness. Avoid the overpriced, promotional "modified" citrus pectin as it has no advantages - except to the people who promote it. Minerals are important here, so include the full complement of calcium, magnesium, boron, zinc, manganese, silicon, chromium, selenium, iodine, iron, vanadium, molybdenum and copper. Curcumin at 500 mg doses is another fine supplement.

Please read my book "Lower Cholesterol Without Drugs" (Safe Goods Publishing) and you will learn things you will never read anywhere else - like how our hormones influence our blood lipids. You must test and balance your basic hormones such as melatonin, testosterone, DHEA, progesterone, estriol, estrone, estradiol, pregnenolone, insulin, T3, T4, and growth hormone in order to keep your cholesterol and triglycerides low and your heart and arterial system healthy.

Topic 9: Breast Health

The three problems most commonly suffered by women in their breasts are cysts, tumors and cancer. The breasts are strongly hormonally influenced, very sensitive and easily susceptible to problems. More than any other organ, especially during puberty, pregnancy and menopause, the breasts are influenced by our endocrine hormones. Estrogens, especially estradiol and estrone, cause cell proliferation and can be the basis of excessive and malignant growth. At Harvard Medical School in Massachusetts (Journal of the National Cancer Institute 90 (1998) p. 1292-99) concluded, "The authors' data in conjunction with past epidemiological and animal studies, provide strong evidence for a causal relationship between postmenopausal estrogen levels and the risk of breast cancer." More proof of this is that women with ovarectomies or hysterectomies (the ovaries always atrophy and die after the uterus is removed) have less breast cancer due to lower estrogen levels. Progesterone, on the other hand, slows and moderates the growth of breast cells and influences them to mature.

Women with normal to high estrogen and low progesterone levels are prime candidates for abnormal breast cell growth due to the RATIO of estrogen to progesterone. Women who are anovulatory (when they don't produce progesterone and are not even aware they aren't), have more breast problems (New England Journal of Medicine 1975, vol. 293, p. 790-5). Research around the world shows over and over that women with low progesterone levels have up to 500% more risk of early breast cancer. Such women also have up to ten times the normal death rate from all malignant neoplasms (cancerous growths) and three times the normal death rate from all causes (American Journal of Epidemiology 1981, vol. 114). Keeping youthful levels of progesterone will also help you to live longer. Women on birth control pills have more breast problems due to excess estrogen from the synthetic and unnatural estrogens in those pills.

Since you have a one in eight chance of getting breast cancer in your life, all women should read Robert Kradjian's book

"Save Yourself from Breast Cancer." He shows that women in industrialized countries generally have about 600% more breast cancer than women in agrarian countries due to high FAT diets. 85% of this occurs after the age of 45 when progesterone levels fall severely and the estrogen to progesterone ratio changes so radically. It takes two to sixteen years for the tumors to grow large enough to be detected during examination. Only in America and the European countries are one eighth of the women coming down with outright breast cancer. This rising epidemic of breast cancer only applies basically to white European affluent countries. This is not a genetic situation as only 6% of identical twins both get breast cancer. In the Journal of the American Medical Association (July 21, 1993) only 2.5% of breast cancer was attributed to family history. So, why is this happening? Our high FAT diet is clearly the main reason here and high fat diets are the single most important factor. There is no other explanation in the world that better explains breast cancer rates than total fat intake - and by total fat intake this means all fats including vegetables oils.

You can prove that to yourself by looking at the following chart which is based on the fat calories eaten by women around the world. The thirteen leading cancer countries all eat about 40% fat calories mostly from animal sources (Cancer Research 1985, vol. 45, p. 615-754). In many Asian and African countries people generally eat ten or fifteen percent fat calories and those mostly of vegetable origin. Migration studies further prove this when these women come to the U.S. and adopt the typical Western diet they get the same high rates as European women. One good example is that only one in every one hundred and twenty women in the country of Kenya get breast cancer - less than one per cent. Less than one in one hundred Kenyan women get breast cancer because they can't afford the luxury of a high fat diet. The death rate in American women has not improved despite the endless propaganda that we are "winning the war on cancer". The fact is it gets worse every year. You can protect yourself from breast and other cancers simply by eating less than twenty per cent fats with most of them coming from vegetables. You will hear of fallacious studies that deny any relationship of dietary fat to breast cancer such as the Harvard Nurses Study. In this study they merely lowered the fat intake from the usual 42% to 32%, which simply didn't make any real difference. You must go under the critical level of 20% and preferably down to 15%. The ideal is 10% total fat calories, which many cultures maintain normally.

Don't think this is only due to saturated animal fats, as some studies show that vegetable oils promote tumor growth just as quickly as animal fats. Always remember that high fat intake equals high estrogen levels equals high breast cancer rates. Instead of listening to the medical propaganda that "early detection is your best protection", realize that PREVENTION is your best protection. PREVENTION IS YOUR BEST PROTECTION. You can PREVENT breast cancer by cutting down or eliminating red meat, poultry, eggs, milk and dairy foods. Women who drink coffee and alcohol also have more breast problems. You are not going to have healthy breasts as long as you drink coffee or alcohol even moderately.

Another strong dietary factor is drinking milk and eating dairy products made from milk including yogurt. The British Journal of Cancer (vol. 61 (1990) p. 456) proved that women who drink milk have many times the lymphoma rate than those who don't. The American Journal of Epidemiology (vol. 130 (1989) p. 904) showed that women milk drinkers also have far more ovarian cancer. There are numerous similar studies showing this.

At the European Institute of Oncology in Milan (Journal of the National Cancer Institute vol. 90 (1998) p. 389-94) a very interesting study was done on 5,157 women to see which factors were correlated with breast cancer rates. They found that alcohol intake, low beta carotene intake, low vitamin E intake and lack of exercise were especially important. They stressed that these four factors were very easy to modify and could thus prevent at least one third of the breast cancer cases in Italy.

A very important supplement in preventing and treating cancer, including breast cancer, is the extract of tumeric known as curcumin. Taking 500 mg of curcumin (not mere tumeric powder) has been shown to be protective against a variety of human cancers and a powerful supplement in treating them. At Columbia University in New York (Prostate vol. 47 (2001) p. 293-303), for example, doctors found that curcumin was very powerful in inhibiting human prostate cancer cells. Prostate cancer is the male equivalent of female breast cancer in many ways and the causes and cures are very parallel. Beta-sitosterol 300 mg (discussed in the previous chapter) has shown benefit in breast cancer and other forms of cancer such as prostate and colon. DIM 200 mg is good for lowering estrogen levels and improving estrogen metabolism so the more potent estrogens are changed into less potent ones.

CoQ10 100 mg is very powerful for breast health. At the University of Texas (Biochemical and Biophysical Research Communications 1994, v. 3) women with breast cancer were given CoQ10 with no other therapy. Unbelievably they all improved with some women actually having no tumors at all after only three months. This is a most important supplement to take.

The hormone melatonin is vital for protecting us against cancer in general and especially in the breast and prostate. At the Medical School of Lodz in Poland doctors said, "Moreover, preliminary results of use of melatonin in the treatment of cancer patients suggest possible therapeutic role for melatonin in human malignancy" (International Journal of Thymology vol. 4 (1996) p. 75-9). The University of Tubingen in Germany studied this situation and published their findings (Wiener Klinische Wochenschraft vol. 109 (1997) p. 722-9). They said, "A progressive decline of pineal melatonin secretion was observed parallel to the growth of primary breast and prostate cancer indicating substitution therapy to be promising." At the Cancer Registry in Norway (British Journal of Cancer vol. 84 (2001) p. 397-9) studies of 15,000 women showed the ones with the lowest levels of melatonin had the highest rates of breast cancer.

DHEA is another hormone that is important in preventing and treating cancer, especially breast cancer. At the famous Johns Hopkins University Oncology Center in Baltimore researchers found a strong relationship with low DHEA in women with breast cancer (Cancer Research vol. 52 (1992) p. 1-4). They found that "The mean serum levels of DHEA among (cancer) cases was 10% lower than among controls" and that there were more extreme differences in women in the top third of DHEA levels compared with women in the bottom third. DHEA can also be too high in women so it must be measured before supplementing.

Other studies have found that women with low progesterone levels suffer from more of every possible breast disorder including mastitis, mastodynia, cysts, fibrocystic breasts, tumors and nodularity (Obstetrics and Gynecology 1979, vol. 54). Some studies found that low progesterone levels are associated with breast cancer (Journal of Reproductive Medicine 1984, vol. 29). One of these studied postmenopausal women and found breast cancer patients were characterized by high estrogen and low progesterone levels (Pharmacy Science 1995, vol. 8, p. 39-45).

On a more positive note researchers have shown pro-gesterone supplementation inhibits the growth of breast tumors and sarcomas (Acta Chir. Scandanavia 1974, vol. 140 and Acta Pathologica Micro. Scandanavia 1975, vol. 83A) One of these studies used a mere 2.5 mg of progesterone applied directly to the breasts in a gel form to improve breast metabolism in less than two weeks (Fertility and Sterility 1995, vol. 63). Using higher, more physiologically normal doses would have surely resulted in even more dramatic effects. Doctors in Buenos Aires (Journal of Steroid Biochemistry 2000, v. 73) proved the beneficial effects of transdermal progesterone on breast metabolism and alleviating cysts.

The Romanian government granted patent #83,933 (1984) for a progesterone cream especially for mammary pathology specifically mastodynia and mastopathy. The German government granted patent (#3,238,984 91983) for a progesterone gel for mammary disorders. If you are experiencing breast problems you can apply your progesterone cream directly to them according to whether you are pre - or postmenopausal.

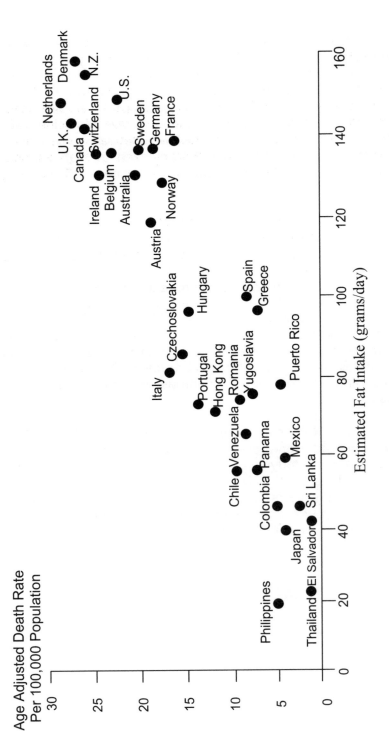

International Breast Cancer Death Rates Related to Fat Intake

Topic 10: A Healthy Uterus and Ovaries

The uterine area is sensitive, very hormonally controlled and subject to many ills - especially fibroids, endometriosis, ovarian cysts, cervical dysplasia, pelvic inflammatory disease (PID), polycystic ovaries and vaginitis. Much of these problems are often due to excessive estrogen levels. Using natural progesterone to balance and oppose these levels can help many of these problems. Never get x-rays as these only add to your risk of cancer and malignancy. Forget the mantra, "early detection is your best protection" and remember that PREVENTION IS YOUR BEST PROTECTION. Getting a safe, inexpensive sonogram (echogram) or a more expensive MRI (magnetic resonance imagery) is always a good idea.

The worst problem, obviously, is outright cancer, and this can be the only real basic justification for such a drastic procedure as a hysterectomy. Have you ever asked yourself if surgically removing your uterus and/or ovaries is really the answer when you have cancer? Did you ever consider that this is just a symptom and you need to look at the cause of what gave you the cancer? High fat diets raise estrogen levels thus causing uterine cancers (Teratogenesis, Carcinogenesis and Mutagenesis 1995, v. 15, p. 167-77). Before you submit yourself for such destructive surgery, radiation and chemotherapy, which will ruin and shorten your life, please go read Milenka Dobic's book "My Beautiful Life". She had uterine cancer and started to get the usual medical treatment. After she met several women who had actually undergone this and saw how terribly they had been damaged she looked for a natural way to treat herself. She stopped eating meat, poultry, eggs, milk, dairy, refined foods, tropical foods and sweeteners. She refused all medications, surgery and radiation. She started eating whole grains, vegetables, beans, salads and fruits, and within one year she was cancer free. She followed the very unnecessarily rigid traditional Japanese style macrobiotic diet, did not take supplements and did not balance her hormones. She would have had a much easier time of it by eating American macrobiotic foods, taking proven supplements and testing and supplementing her basic hormones. This is a true story of a woman no different from you, and she did cure ovarian cancer in only one year. She did this simply with changing what she ate and making better food choices. This is an inspiring story you should read before you blindly let doctors get hold of you. Always remember that your ovaries atrophy and die after a hysterectomy even though your doctor rarely will tell you that. If you have uterine, ovarian or any other type of cancer consider using progesterone even if you choose the traditional medical route of surgery, radiation and chemotherapy. Studies have also shown potential here in other types of cancers such as renal and kidney cancer (Journal of Steroid Biochemistry 1976).

Fibroids (aka myomas) are benign tumors composed of muscle and fibrous tissue that can grow to the size of grapefruits. Fortunately only about 1 in 200 women will develop malignant fibroids. A simple ultrasound (sonogram) test will reveal these. These develop most often when women are in their thirties. After menopause, as estrogen levels fall the fibroids generally stop growing. Some estimates are that 80% of American women will develop fibroids. Black women develop about 50% more and Asian women develop less than Caucasian women. Fibroids often cause the uterus to drop, which, in turn, causes urinary incontinence. Women with heavy, painful and irregular periods are most at risk here for fibroid growth. These are almost impossible to remove even by the most advanced laser surgery since they are composed of muscle and fiber mixed together and are actually part of the uterus. Prescription drugs are ineffective. Using natural progesterone can help stop their growth, but shrinking them is very difficult. Improving the progesterone to estrogen ratio is simply not enough, and you have to lower your estradiol and estrone to shrink them. A low fat, high fiber, low calorie basically vegetarian diet is the most effective way to do this. Supplement recommended here would be DIM 200 mg (di-indolylmethane), and flax oil 2 g, which lower estrogen levels and improve estrogen metabolism. These are discussed in the supplements chapter. Beta-sitosterol in 300 mg doses has been shown to benefit uterine functioning (Biochemical Molecular Biological International 1993, v. 31, p. 659-68). Losing weight, not eating saturated fats, avoiding alcohol and getting more exercise are good ways to lower high estrogen levels. There are two more specific ways to shrink fibroids and that is to fast (on water only) for two to four weeks at a health center, or go on a very low calorie diet permanently. Read either of Roy Walford's two books on calorie restriction "The 120 Year Diet" and "Maximum Lifespan." Fibroids are simply not a justification for something as drastic as a hysterectomy, although this is done all the time.

Endometriosis occurs when pieces of the uterine lining grow outside the uterus in nearby inappropriate place. These pieces of tissue migrate into the uterus and Fallopian tubes, to the ovaries and even into the colon. This can cause excruciating pain, which is worse during menstruation, as these pieces then bleed. Since these are actual endometrial tissues they swell with blood and bleed. Again, this is a modern disease that does not seem to be known a hundred years ago, as the symptoms were not in the medical literature. One major cause is high estrogen and low progesterone levels (Chiba Igaku Zasshi 19993, v. 69, p. 269-74). This is very difficult to diagnose except by laproscopy (surgical insertion of a tiny medical camera). This condition also tends to cease at menopause due to lower estrogen levels. Progesterone can be very helpful here as is the lowering of estrogen levels.

Ovarian cysts are caused by failed or disordered ovulation and cause abdominal pain. This is getting to be an epidemic in Western countries and many women do not know they have them. These occur mostly in the thirties. Sonograms will show whether a cyst exists and whether it is benign or malignant. Surgery is the usual medical treatment and can result in the loss of one or both ovaries. Natural progesterone used days 12 to 26 of your cycle (day 1 is the first day of your period) suppresses luteinizing hormone (LH) and has stimulating effects that benefit the ovaries. Healthy diet, natural supplements and hormone balancing are a much safer approach to an ovarian cyst. This can be cured naturally with a healthy diet the same way outright cancer can be. Surgery should always be the last option.

Cervical dysplasia is abnormal growth of cervical cells due to the papilloma virus, and is a pre-cancerous condition that can quickly lead to malignancy. This is very common now and is medically treated by a variety of allopathic surgical procedures resulting in permanent damage to the cervix and even sterility. Freezing the surface of the cervix and cone biopsies mutilate the opening and the infection reoccurs. Even symptomatic treatment with topical retinoic acid (Journal American Academy of Dermatology 1986, p. 826-9) is a better choice, but few doctors are even that informed. This is still allopathic and removes the symptom without addressing the cause. A much more sensible approach is eating whole, natural low-fat foods, and avoiding dairy products, meat, poultry and eggs. Use natural progesterone applied to your abdomen (International Journal of Cancer 1992, v. 52, p. 247-51). Take vitamin B-6, vitamin E, beta carotene, folic acid, beta sitosterol, magnesium, beta glucan, curcumin, CoQ10, DIM and other supplements to strengthen your immune system. Balance all your basic hormones by first testing your levels. If you are on birth control pills or estrogen supplements talk with your doctor about getting off these. The Pill is a major factor here. This condition can be cured naturally in 90 days without drugs or surgery. As always, the real cure is eating better foods. There is just no reason to resort to surgery when this can be effectively cured with diet and supplements.

PID (aka salpingitis) is a serious bacterial inflammation of the uterus and Fallopian tubes that can result in permanent damage. Antibiotics and surgery are the usual allopathic treatments. Natural progesterone and an intravaginal estriol cream can be helpful here along with the usual better diet, supplements and hormone balancing. You should test all three of your estrogen levels. Medical doctors are unfamiliar with estriol and regular pharmacies do not carry it. Do not use estriol unless you test for it and determine your levels are low.

Polycystic ovary syndrome (PCOS) is very common now in Western countries and is characterized by many small surface ovarian cysts. The eggs stay on the surface and form a cyst rather than be released. One cause of this is vascular impedence (reduced blood flow to the ovaries). Obesity is often a factor, but is not necessarily a factor. Usually women have high LH, prolactin, testosterone and androstenedione levels and sometimes high DHEA levels, as well as the usual estrogen dominance from estradiol and estrone and low progesterone levels. High triglycerides, a negative blood fat profile and high cardiovascular risk also tend to characterize PCOS. You definitely want to get an accurate, safe and inexpensive sonogram as there may be no

36

symptoms. This is the most common single cause of menstrual irregularity. Insulin resistance is closely connected and must be determined with a GTT (glucose tolerance test). In fact, insulin resistance is almost synonymous with PCOS. Since insulin resistance is also epidemic (see Topic 13: Progesterone and Diabetes) in Western countries, a routine GTT is always a good idea. Progesterone can be of great help here as well as 800 IU of vitamin D. Treat insulin resistance as you would diabetes with a total program of diet, supplements and natural hormone balance.

Vaginitis is an imbalance of the vaginal flora, is very common and can be uncomfortable and embarrassing. It is often caused by birth control pills or estrogen supplements. This is usually treated medically with powerful antibiotics that only make the natural balance of the beneficial vaginal bacteria worse. If you are on birth control pills or estrogen supplements speak with your doctor about getting off of these. Very good diet, natural progesterone cream, proven supplements and intravaginal estriol cream (you must test your estriol level first) can be of great help. Many studies for decades now have shown the value of using an estriol vaginal gel for menopause and vaginal atrophy (Maturitas 1981 v. 3, p. 321-7). You must also get this from a compounding pharmacist. You can consider herbal douches here, but no more than once a week or you'll upset the natural balance in your vagina.

You cannot get estriol cream except from a compounding pharmacist. If you cannot find one in your town you can contact the Professional Compounding Centers of America or the International Academy of Compounding Pharmacists:

PCCA   IACP
   (800) 331-2498   (800) 927-4227

Uterine Cancer is Due to Fat Intake

Incidence of uterine
cancer / 100,000 women

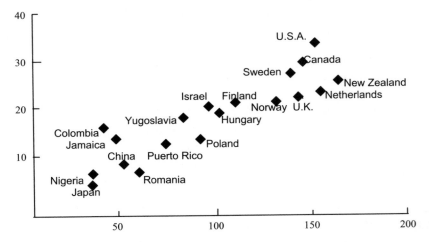

PER CAPITA DAILY TOTAL FAT CONSUMPTION – GRAMS

Decreasing follicles mean less progesterone

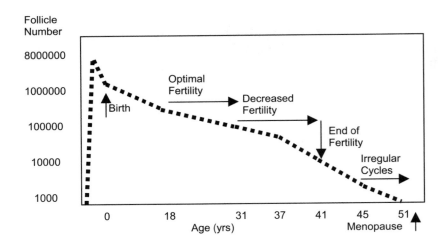

Topic 11: PMS- Premenstrual Syndrome

The occurrence of physical and psychological changes in women during the week prior to the onset of their periods dates back to the time of Hippocrates, the "father of medicine", over 2000 years ago. PMS is now estimated to occur in two thirds of American women. Ironically, it can be rare in poor, agrarian countries. It is a complex condition with multiple causes including hormones, nutrients, social and psychological factors. The most common complaints are irritability (almost universal), emotional instability, tension, and headaches. There are no single deficiencies or excesses which can be consistently identified. The best way to deal with a complicated problem like this is basically with diet, supplements, hormone balancing, not taking prescription drugs, exercising and avoiding bad habits. A good example is at the University of Colorado (J. Repro. Med. 1987, v.32, p. 405-22) women were given better diets with less meat and dairy and more complex carbohydrates and vegetables. In addition they were given vitamin and mineral supplements. This regimen resulted in very strong reduction in premenstrual problems. A very fine group of doctors, including Neal Barnard and Dean Ornish, formed the Physicians Committee for Responsible Medicine (PCRM) to advocate natural health practices. They published a study (Obstetrics and Gynecology 95 (2000) p. 245-50) where 33 women were fed a low-fat, vegetarian diet for two menstrual cycles. These women lost weight, their menstrual cycles improved and their PMS symptoms lessened. These simple changes lowered their estrogen levels and had many other beneficial effects.

Seven to ten days prior to a woman's cycle, in the luteal phase (the twelve days prior to the period), various physical and psychological symptoms appear. These increase in intensity as the mense approaches and then cease with the onset or slightly after the start. In the luteal phase progesterone is not normally low, but has been found to be so in some, but not all, women. There is a very strong hormonal factor here generally, but it is not yet well understood. It is important to test your estradiol, estrone, estriol, DHEA, progesterone, testosterone, pregnenolone, thyroid and melatonin levels and balance them accordingly. You can also test your cortisol level to see if you are under undue stress, but it is very difficult to lower high cortisol levels except by exercise and lifestyle. A GTT (glucose tolerance) test for insulin is good, too.

It is rather amazing, but over 60 years ago, Dr. Leon Israel (J. Amer. Med. Assoc. 110 (1938) p. 1721-3) found that during this time "only" 40% of women complained of "premenstrual tension." He said this was largely caused by low progesterone and could be remedied very effectively with injections of natural progesterone. Remember this was before the invention of synthetic progestins, and the only progesterone available was real human progesterone. He treated these women with very expensive progesterone (extracted from corpses) with good success. Over 60 years later we are finally realizing he was right. Doctors at the time were doing hysterectomies by beaming intense radiation directly at the uterus in order to destroy it, instead of operating and surgically removing it! Obviously this led to many horrible side effects, especially outright cancer, and this practice was stopped. Doctors try and hide such facts today just as 50 years from now they will try to hide the fact one third of American women get unnecessary hysterectomies. At the time (1938) Dr. Israel described the main symptoms of "premenstrual tension" as tense irritability, crying, headache, vertigo, insomnia, restlessness, painful breasts, nymphomania(!), dysmenorrhea, and stomatitis.

Progesterone can be a help to some women, but by itself this is not a panacea (cure all) by any means. Katharina Dalton claimed an 83% success rate in improving symptoms of PMS in 86 women (Can. J. Psychiat. 30 (1985), p. 483-7) who were given high doses of natural progesterone during their luteal phase. She has worked with over 30,000 women and started her work almost 50 years ago. While this sounds promising, other researchers did not get such positive results and the issue is far more complicated than simply progesterone levels prior to menses.

Diet should be the focus here as it should be in any illness. A study at the University of Colorado (cited earlier) studied the dietary intake of women who suffered PMS regularly. These women consumed 275% more refined sugar and sweeteners, 62% more refined carbohydrates (instead of whole grains) and 79% more dairy products, 78% more sodium, 52% less zinc, 77%

40

less magnesium, 53% less iron, half the fiber and drank more coffee than the healthy women. Also, their source of fats and proteins were mainly from animal sources rather than vegetable sources. Women who eat more fat, especially saturated animal fat have higher blood levels of estrogens than women who eat 20% or less fat calories. The doctors suggested women with PMS cut down greatly on simple sugars, eat more whole complex carbohydrates, eat more fiber (whole grains and beans are the best sources of fiber), and eat less meat, poultry, eggs and dairy products. This means less calorie intake and less obesity. They also suggested supplementing with all minerals especially magnesium, iron, zinc and manganese, as well as vitamin A (use 25,000 IU of beta carotene instead), B-6, C and E. Flax oil would be a better source of the essential fatty acids they recommended rather than primrose oil.

Probably the most enlightening study ever published on this was by Kathleen Head in the Alternative Medicine Review (volume 2 (1997) p. 12-25). After extensively reviewing this complex set of symptoms we call PMS she found women could be divided into four basic types, even though they often included the symptoms of two different types.

PMT-A was the most common type and affects over two-thirds of American women. Here mental and emotional symptoms dominate with anxiety, depression, irritability, insomnia and generalized nervous tension occurring. In PMT-A estrogen clearly dominates progesterone and there is a lack of physical symptoms. For PMT-A natural progesterone therapy seems very promising.

PMT-H was the second most common type affecting less than two-thirds of American women. This is a very physical condition with weight gain, abdominal bloating, tender and engorged breasts and edema (water retention) in the face, hands and feet. They found low dopamine levels generally in these women.

PMT-C occurs in less than a quarter of the women and is clearly related to blood sugar metabolism and pre-diabetic symptoms. Such women should treat this type as if they had diabetes and eat a diet based on whole grains and vegetables with no fruits, fruit juice, dried fruit, sugars or sweets of any kind. The symptoms here are increased appetite, craving for sweet foods (especially chocolate), symptoms of hypoglycemia including headaches, fainting, fatigue, dizziness, palpitations and trembling. High insulin levels were shown here thru GTT testing.

PMT-D was least common, rarely occurred alone, was harder to define, and occurred in less than five per cent of the women, more or less, but more frequently when combined with PMT-A. This type more often occurs in combination with PMT-A and is characterized by depression, lethargy, sadness, crying, confusion, gloom, a sense of hopelessness and helplessness and even suicidal tendencies in a minority of subjects. Here we find a very unusual predominance of progesterone over estrogen, so progesterone therapy is clearly not indicated at all.

Medical doctors will often be unsympathetic here and not realize the biological basis of much of this. Diuretics are offered for symptoms such as water retention. These are just more examples of trying to cover up the symptom while ignoring the underlying cause. Obviously estrogen supplements, especially horse estrogen, estradiol or estrone will just make most women worse. These are nearly always prescribed without first determining whether estrogen levels are low in the first place. Giving synthetic progestins have none of the benefits of natural progesterone and have many side effects including lowering actual progesterone levels and making PMS symptoms worse (Acta. Endoctin. Kabenh. 66 (1971), p. 799). Doctors will very often prescribe antidepressants and anti-anxiety agents such as Prozac, Xanax, Zoloft or Valium and refuse to deal with the many possible causes of these very real symptoms. Some doctors actually go as far as to recommend a complete hysterectomy (and remember your ovaries die even if they are not removed) to treat PMS! More enlightened doctors like Guy Abraham (J. Appl. Nutr. 36 (1984), p. 103-24) are aware of the literature on PMS and the groupings of it into four basic categories. For PMT-A he suggested strong doses of vitamin B-6 (megadoses of any supplement are always wrong), mineral supplements, eating more fiber, eating less dairy and animal products, using less sweets and applying natural progesterone. For PMT-H he again suggests vitamin B-6 in high doses (however, more than 10 mg is harmful long term) and avoiding caffeine, nicotine and alcohol completely. For PMT-C he recommends magnesium, fatty acids (use flax oil), avoiding all sweets and getting a glucose tolerance test. For PMT-D this is much harder to treat and a complete physical with comprehensive hormone testing is called for, possible high toxic metal levels in the blood, and psychiatric counseling if severe depression or suicidal thoughts are present.

A good study from the University of Calgary (Clin. Invest. Med. 20 (1997) p. 211-23) gave oral progesterone supplements to women with PMS during their luteal phase and got good general improvement. If they had used transdermal progesterone certainly the results would have been better, as oral progesterone requires very high doses and is mostly broken down into unwanted metabolites. At the Institute of Endokrinology in Moscow women with edema complaints prior to their menses were found to be low in progesterone (Probl. Endokrinol. 25 (1979), p. 32-6). At the University of Umea in Sweden (J. Ster. Biochem. 5, (1974), p. 257-60) women with PMT-A symptoms were found to be low in progesterone, high in estrogen, and gaining body weight during the last of their periods. Doctors at the Institute of Endocrinology in Prague found women with PMS symptoms generally had low levels of progesterone in the follicular phase (the time of the cycle after the period) of their cycles as compared to controls without such symptoms (Horm. Metabl Res. (30 (1998) p. 227-30).

Katharina Dalton writing almost 50 years ago (Brit. Med. J. May 9, 1953, p. 1007-14) noted then that "only" about 40% of women complained about premenstrual problems compared with over 70% today. This is very significant to see such an increase. The term at the time was "premenstrual tension." Katharina was a real pioneer in women's health and her studies are still quoted today. She noted that as far back as 1937 it was known that excessive estrogen levels caused water retention - one of the classic signs of PMS. She said, "The concept of an abnormally high oestradiol/progesterone (the English spell estradiol as "oestradiol") ratio has much in its support." Notice the word "ratio" as a woman can have either high estrogen or low progesterone levels or both. She reviewed earlier work in the 1940's where doctors had successfully treated women with PMS by injecting them with natural progesterone. Please remember that synthetic progestins had not yet been invented and the idea of transdermal progesterone was simply not discovered. She was also trying to use testosterone therapy for the women, but the only forms used by doctors at the time were unnatural oral salts and esters and not natural testosterone gels and creams. Nor did she test the women for testosterone levels. Her success with progesterone injections were stunning and now being "rediscovered" a half century later.

Why would a physician give a woman unnatural progestins instead of real, natural progesterone? A study done at PMS Medical in New York (Comprehensive Therapy 19 (1993) p. 96-8) showed that women given synthetic progestins worsened their PMS symptoms. If they had been given natural progesterone as a supplement their symptoms would have clearly improved. Some doctors will actually give women these progestins and call them "progesterone", thus leading their patients to believe this is actually real progesterone. This is criminal. Taking progestins actually decreases the production of biological progesterone by the body making the blood levels even lower.

Medical doctors rarely understand that hormones are a major factor in PMS, but this has been published internationally and is common knowledge in clinical studies. Melatonin, for example, is very important here. Doctors at the University of California in La Jolla (Journal of Biological Rhythms 12 (1997) p. 47-64) showed that women suffering from symptoms before their periods generally had low melatonin levels. They said, "These findings replicate the author's previous observation that nocturnal melatonin concentrations are decreased in with PMDD (premenstrual dysphoric disorder)".

Some herbs, especially chaste tree (Vitex agnus castus), dong quai, black cohosh (be careful with this one), blue cohosh and alfalfa extract may be helpful. Everyone is biologically different and one herb may help one person yet be toxic to another, so only trial and error can help you here. Doctors in Germany (Phytomed. 4 (1997) p. 183-9) in a placebo controlled study gave both 100 mg of vitamin B-6 (don't take more than 10 mg long term) and chaste tree extract to women with PMS and got good results with both. Researchers at United Medical School in London (Curr. Top. Nutr. Dis. 19 (1988), p. 363-79) also found that giving women high doses (you can only tolerate high does for about 90 days) of vitamin B-6, especially when combined with magnesium supplements, gave good response for PMS symptoms. The reason pyridoxine (B-6) stands out is that it is important in the synthesis of dopamine and serotonin - two very important metabolic regulators and are involved in depression (Vitamins and Hormones 36 (1978) p. 53-99). The RDA for B-6 is only 2 mg a day so 10 mg is a good long term dose. Megadoses, even of water soluble vitamins, are harmful in the long term. Use such doses only for a week prior to your period temporarily. More doctors in Germany (Brit. Med. J. 322 (2001), p. 134-7) studied 170 women with PMS and gave them the equivalent of two 500 mg capsules of chaste tree and got over half the women to respond well in a placebo controlled study. Please notice that half did not respond, since herbal remedies are just not universal. Other published studies found the same basic results in an herb that has been known for over 2,000 years now. Taking all the supplements recommended in the "Natural Supplements" chapter will go a long way to raise your immunity, improve your metabolism, and raise your general level of health so you will be successfully and effectively dealing with the very complex and not well understood myriad causes of PMS.

If you are on prescription drugs or birth control pills talk to your doctor about getting off for at least three months to see if there is any improvement. Get off them permanently if you want to be healthy. Most any medications may cause or make PMS symptoms worse. Obviously you'll be far better off with a natural alternative to your prescription drug whatever it is. You are never going to enjoy good health while taking some toxic, unnatural, synthetic prescription chemical with dangerous side effects that covers up your symptoms while worsening the underlying cause.

Exercise is the most important aspect of lifestyle next to diet. Women athletes and women who exercise regularly show far less PMS than other women. In Finland women who participated in sports had far less PMS symptoms that women who didn't exercise at all (Acta. Obstet. Gynecol. Scand. 50 (1971) p. 331). Alcohol intake is more harmful to women than men and often upsets their reproductive systems. Women are simply much more sensitive to even one alcoholic drink a day. Just one or two drinks daily can cause serious medical problems in women. Alcohol is shown to inhibit proper glucose metabolism and blood sugar levels. Coffee has become a national addiction in the last few years and coffee consumption will make your symptoms worse. Caffeine intake is just not good, especially for women, and has been shown to be correlated with breast cysts and other breast diseases. The unfiltered, espresso, Turkish and French press coffees that contain the oils that filters take out are much more harmful than filtered coffee. Smoking may well be connected with PMS and it is well connected with such problems as premature menopause, osteoporosis and coronary heart disease. One third of American women smoke cigarettes. If you exercise regularly, stop drinking alcohol, stop smoking, and don't drink coffee you'll have a much better chance of being symptom free every month. Healthy women really are symptom free and don't suffer these problems every month prior to their periods - there is nothing natural, normal or inherent in suffering every cycle. The menstrual cycle is by nature a healthy one without any negative symptoms. The unpleasant experiences most women suffer every month between the ages of 13 and 52 are due to less than ideal health. Many women go thru life experiencing their cycles with no problems at all, especially in poor Third World countries where they work hard by necessity and cannot afford the luxuries of a high fat, refined diet with too many calories. American women eat twice the calories they need, half the fiber they need, five times the fat they need, twice the protein they need and 125 pounds of sweeteners they have no need of at all. This is on top of the refined foods, chemicals, preservatives, coffee, alcohol and nicotine. Add stress to this and you can understand the epidemic rates of most every known medical condition and disease in American women.

Topic 12: How to Use Progesterone

The most convenient, practical and effective way to use natural progesterone is with transdermal (through the skin) cream or gel. Some hormones like progesterone, estradiol, estrone, estriol and testosterone readily penetrate the skin into the fat cells and then into our bloodstreams. Injections are painful, difficult, unnatural, expensive and very unnecessary. Anal or vaginal suppositories are far less convenient than transdermal cream. A nasal spray is very practical, but would have to be approved by the FDA and sold only by prescription at high cost unfortunately. The various oral and sublingual (under the tongue) preparations use very large amounts of progesterone, which break down into unwanted metabolites as it is digested. This problem with taking real progesterone orally is due to the fact it is broken down by the liver after it leaves the stomach. NEVER take oral progesterone no matter what claims are made for it. A good transdermal cream avoids this problem by putting it right into your bloodstream.

We have already discussed women who take birth control pills and why they should use progesterone. We have also discussed women who have had hysterectomies. Using progesterone is very different for pre- and postmenopausal women.

If you are still having periods always cycle this with your period from day 12 to day 26 (day 1 is the first day of your period). This is the natural way to parallel your cycle and the way your body produces progesterone. This way you are using a natural hormone in a natural way. Just apply some for two weeks from day 12 to 26. A half teaspoon of cream containing, say, 1000 mg per two ounce jar will give you about 33 mg on your skin. Of this, at least 20-25 mg will penetrate your skin and go into your bloodstream. This is about the amount you would normally produce each day during this two-week part of your cycle. A jar will last about two months using it this way.

If you are no longer having periods just use a quarter teaspoon every day any three weeks of the calendar month. Give

47

yourself one week off each month. A two ounce jar will last over two months when used this way. You will do this the rest of your life and benefit greatly from it.

If you have a specific problem like fibrocystic breasts or endometriosis you can apply the cream directly to the area that is affected. Always apply this to soft, thin tissue and not thick areas of skin. Breasts, abdomen, inner thighs, and inner wrists are all soft thin tissue that the progesterone penetrates well. If you apply this to thick skin like stomach or arms the progesterone will basically penetrate the skin and tend to stay in the fat cells rather than entering the bloodstream. There is no need to use larger amounts with the idea that "more is better". You are looking for a natural balance of estrogens and progesterone, and not for excessive levels of any hormone no matter how beneficial.

If you want your progesterone levels tested you can go to a medical doctor and have him draw blood and send it to a laboratory. This is expensive and requires an office visit and most doctors are very unfamiliar with hormone testing and hormone levels strangely enough. What do they go to medical school for? If you do have a blood test be sure to insist on a serum test and not a plasma test, as progesterone is fat soluble and measuring serum is much more accurate. A much more practical and less expensive way is to use saliva testing from one of the labs mentioned in the chapter on Home Hormone Testing. Saliva testing gives unbound, bioavailable levels and can be done in the privacy of your home for as little as $25 or $30. It is very important to note that progesterone testing must be done at specific times of your cycle if you are still menstruating.

Progesterone transdermal creams are usually sold in two ounce jars or tubes and should contain 800 to 1,000 mg of USP natural micronized progesterone per jar (400 to 500 mg per ounce in other words). Never, never, never buy any cream with the words "yam", "wild yam", "Mexican yam" etc. on the label, as this is known as "yam scam" in the trade. Yam extract does NOT convert to progesterone in the body and is NOT a precursor biologically. The confusion comes from the fact that biochemical laboratories do use yam and soy extracts as raw materials when they produce progesterone by sophisticated and elaborate chemical manufacturing processes.

Remember that the production of progesterone goes from about 20 mg a day to about 400 mg a day during pregnancy - a 2,000% rise! So, there is a wide latitude for safety. Progesterone is very safe and non-toxic with no known side effects, especially when the most that will be used is a half teaspoon of cream (about 33 mg) two weeks per month. Women who are still having periods should be assured their estrogen levels are sufficient or they wouldn't be able to menstruate. Any doctor that wants to give you synthetic progestins instead of real natural progesterone, or wants to give you estradiol or estrone without testing your levels is telling you he is not competent to treat you - or anyone else. Women who are taking horse estrogen, estradiol or estrone should cut back slowly over a three month period to get off them. After you are off all estrogen supplements for at least one month you can have your free levels of estradiol, estrone and estriol tested to prove that your levels are sufficient. The fact is that most women in America have too much estrogen from fat intake, obesity, alcohol use, lack of exercise and other factors, so that estrogen supplements make an already bad situation even worse. You'll notice that your doctor is probably not even aware of the third estrogen which is estriol. This is considered the "safe" or good estrogen. Ironically, no pharmaceutical company in America even manufactures it nor normal pharmacies sell it! It comprises more than 80% of your total blood estrogen level yet doctors and pharmacists generally know nothing of it! If your levels test low you can obtain this from a compounding pharmacist as a vaginal cream or gel. Try using a half gram daily of a 0.3% mixture and 100 grams will last you almost seven months. Estriol has been called "the forgotten estrogen", but most all the saliva testing laboratories are well aware of it and know how to test your levels.

Besides progesterone and the three basic estrogens, it is important to realize that our endocrine (ductless glands that secrete our hormones) system is a united system. No hormone works alone; all our hormones work in concert together and work best when they are at youthful levels - neither too high nor too low. In the chapter "Natural Hormone Balance" you'll read more about your other basic hormones, what they are, and how to test and balance them for optimum health. Along with using natural progesterone you should also make sure you have a youthful DHEA level. DHEA can be either too high or too low but in people over 40 it is usually low. Testosterone is important for women even though they only have one-tenth the amount that men do. In women testosterone can either be too high or too low, so you must test your level. Pregnenolone is the most important of all hormones that affects our brain and is the "grandmother" hormone. Women over 40 are usually low in this and can get a blood test done for about $150 or find one of the very few saliva testing labs that are testing for this. Melatonin is the "anti-aging" hormone and is vital to every system in our body. Melatonin actually has strong anti-cancer properties among many other benefits. Our levels of this fall from the time we leave our teenage years. Cortisol is usually too high in women in the industrialized countries, but can only be changed through lifestyle. Growth hormone can be measured with a blood test for about $100 as no saliva testing lab is currently offering this service. The only way to raise growth hormone is through injections of actual recombinant human growth hormone at a cost of about $300 to $500 a month. The thyroid hormones T3 and T4 should be tested by either blood or saliva. You can use human equivalent T3 and T4 hormones (Cytomel and Syntroid), but you must test and use these separately. You can get your insulin tested with a simple glucose tolerance test (GTT) to see if your insulin is too high due to insulin resistance. Both thyroid and insulin problems are epidemic in Americans over the age of 50.

It is interesting that doctors rarely test your hormones even when prescribing potent estradiol, estrone and horse estrogens. One would logically think that medical doctors would routinely check all the basic hormones we have just discussed, but they rarely do. Now you have a choice of having your doctor do this, or using a saliva test kit for most of your hormones. Soon we will have saliva testing for all the hormones and won't need to go to doctors to get this done. Always remember that these hormones all work together in concert and should all be balanced at youthful levels as much as possible. Progesterone is a very beneficial hormone, but is only one part of the endocrine picture and has the greatest benefits when supported by all the others.

Topic 13: Progesterone and Diabetes

Progesterone in our bodies helps to normalize blood sugar and insulin levels. Diabetes is an epidemic in our country with 800,000 new cases a year now affecting over 16 million people. Every year more and more and younger people are diagnosed with it. Insulin resistance is even more of an epidemic and not as obvious. This occurs when excess insulin is produced as the cells are no longer reacting effectively to it. Since 1990 the rate of new cases has risen over 40%. What are these epidemics due to? For starters, our extreme intake of over 150 pounds of various sweeteners, our fat intake, which is almost half of our calories, our protein intake which is twice what we need, the refined foods we eat, and the fact we eat twice the calories we need. Over 90% of this is type II, which is due to dysmetabolism of insulin. In type I there is not enough insulin produced by the pancreas. The causative factors are AGE, obesity, lack of exercise, family genetics and race. Medical doctors tell us this is "incurable" and prescribe oral or injected prescription drugs for the rest of the person's life. It is the seventh leading cause of death in the U.S. Diabetes eventually results in early death, amputation of limbs, blindness, kidney failure and various forms of heart disease. The symptoms are usually lack of energy, chronic tiredness, and physical weakness even after sleep or naps. You should get your blood sugar levels tested along with a glucose tolerance test (GTT). Anyone over 30 should get a GTT to test their insulin level as doctors almost never recommend this.

Back in 1972 it was discovered that progesterone increased insulin effectiveness (Endocrinology vol. 91, p. 77-81). In 1974 diabetes was controlled in laboratory animals with just progesterone supplementation (Hormone Metabolism Research vol. 6, p. 4301). Other such studies have appeared since then in various medical journals, but neither the medical profession nor the general public has any idea that this research has been done. This is the only published book you will ever find out about these studies and the benefits of progesterone supplementation for diabetes and insulin normalization.

If you have abnormal blood sugar or insulin levels - whether too high or too low - progesterone is a supplement you should be using along with a totally sugar-free diet. This means no sweeteners of any kind no matter how "natural". All simple sugars are basically the same whether you are talking about white sugar, brown sugar, raw sugar, molasses, honey, maple syrup, maltose, fructose, sucrose, corn syrup, amazake, stevia or whatever. If your blood sugar metabolism is abnormal you should no longer eat fresh fruit, dried fruit, fruit juice or anything at all that is sweet, because your body is unable to digest and metabolize it properly. This may sound somewhat extreme but it is necessary. Please realize there is little nutrition in fruit anyway, and most all fruits are just sugar and water with very little vitamin or mineral content at all. Read my "Zen Macrobiotics for Americans" for more on this.

The other thing you should do is take excess fat out of your diet, especially saturated fat. Whenever you study diabetes you almost always find abnormal cholesterol and triglyceride levels - they go hand in hand. Stop eating all red meat, poultry, eggs, and especially dairy products, regardless of how low fat or no fat they are. Remember that dairy products contain indigestible lactose. Eat a plant-based diet with seafood if you have no seafood or fish allergies. Eat very little vegetable oils, and remember that olive oil is not "good for you" no matter what you've been reading. Eat all the whole grains, green and yellow vegetables, beans, soups and salads you want. These digest and metabolize very slowly and normalize your blood sugar levels over time. You can slowly wean yourself off any medications you are taking by sticking to your diet and taking specific supplements. A May 2001 study in the New England Journal of Medicine showed great improvement in diabetics by simply making better food choices, exercising and losing weight.

A perfect example of this is the Pima Indians in Arizona and Mexico. These people all came from the same Pima stock centuries ago, but they now live very different lives. The Pimas in Mexico are slim, generally very healthy and have very little heart disease or diabetes. They live on a traditional diet of corn, beans, vegetables and other natural foods and do not eat much meat, sugar or refined foods, as this is not part of their culture. The Pimas in Arizona are overweight, have numerous health problems, high cholesterol levels and heart disease and high rates of diabetes. They eat a typical American diet of meat, sugar, refined foods and other typical such fare. This is real world proof that complex carbohydrates help prevent diabetes while simple carbohydrates combined with lots of fat help cause diabetes.

The allopathic medical treatments, of course, just address the symptoms and not the cause by prescribing oral or injected insulin. There are very serious side effects to these drugs including severe liver damage, deadly buildup of lactic acid in your blood, acute kidney damage and many other side effects.

This is also real world proof that the "ketogenic diet", "glycemic index" as well as the "Paleolithic diet" don't work, since excess fat is a major cause of diabetes. It is interesting that the author of best selling books on this kind of diet himself suffers from high cholesterol levels, heart disease, blood sugar disorders and other such illnesses. He rarely appears in public anymore since he looks so bad for his age and just was hospitalized for cardiomyopathy! Such books have sold by the millions, because they tell people what they want to hear, rather than what they need to hear.

Diet is the real way to cure abnormal blood sugar and insulin metabolism whether it is diabetes or hypoglycemia. There are herbs and supplements that will help you. All minerals are vital here especially chromium, selenium and vanadium. Search the Internet under "mineral supplements" to find a complete one.

Taking CoQ10 100 mg is important. Alpha lipoic acid has shown value and you should take 200 mg a day. Herbs can only be used for 6 to 12 months and their effects wear off. Ginseng (not Siberian "ginseng" which is unrelated) has also shown effectiveness and you can take two 500 mg capsules of a reliable brand. The herb Gymnema sylvestre may help you and you can take two 500 mg capsules of that. A third herb Momorida charantia (bitter melon) can be taken in the same amounts. A fourth herb is extract of common fenugreek seeds and you can also use two capsules of that. Recently banaba leaf extract from the Lagerstroemia speciosa plant (containing corosolic acid) has been promoted for helping diabetics, but there is little good scientific evidence on this yet. Curcumin (tumeric extract) can be of value and is a fine antioxidant supplement to take anyway. You need about 250 mg of actual curcumoids. Nopal cactus may be of value but there are no studies on this yet. Aloe vera gel can be taken orally every day for one year and may have other good effects. Glutathione metabolism may play a part and glutathione levels can easily be raised by taking NAC (N-acetyl cysteine) supplements 600 mg, which is discussed in the supplements chapter. Vitamin E is an important vitamin here and you can take 400 IU of mixed tocopherols. Beta glucan 200 mg (400 mg for the first six months) is an important supplement to normalize blood sugar levels. Please read my book "What Is Beta Glucan?"

Hormone imbalances are usually found in diabetics. It is vital you get all your basic hormone levels tested and balance them as much as possible. This has been discussed constantly throughout the book. There is so much we don't know about hormone levels and diabetes, so be sure to use natural progesterone and test the levels of all your other important hormones as a foundation for whatever else you do. You'll notice that no doctor talks about hormonal influence in diabetes, nor do the foundations that are supposedly trying to find a cure for it. The studies are right there in the medical journals for all to see.

Most diabetics are overweight and they simply aren't going to get well until getting their weight down to normal. If you eat the foods advised in the natural diet chapter you can eat all you want and lose weight until you are at your ideal size. Please read my book "Zen Macrobiotics for Americans" to learn more about making better food choices. Exercise is very important. If you want to cure diabetes, you are going to have to exercise, even if it is just walking for a half hour a day. Unfortunately, diabetics are unable to fast (on water only) for more than a few hours without getting ill. As you get stronger you'll find you can go longer and longer without any food with no ill effects or discomfort. This shows you are getting better. When you are off all medications you can fast for 24 hours and go longer and longer if there are no problems. Diabetes can be cured within one or two years with good diet, supplements, exercise and hormone balancing with results being seen every month.

Topic 14: Natural Diet

Diet is everything. Nothing is more important to your health than what you eat every day. Your daily food is paramount to your well being. We are literally what we eat. Americans eat twice the calories they need, over six times the fat they need, 150 pounds of various sugars they don't need at all, half the necessary fiber, and twice the necessary protein, yet they are chronically undernourished and lacking in vital nutrients, vitamins and minerals. Let's look at the basic food groups and see what we have available to eat and what is best for us.

Animal flesh such as beef, pork and lamb are very high in saturated fats, very high in calories, contain no fiber and have a very unbalanced profile of nutrients. High consumption of meats is associated with such diseases as diabetes, heart and artery disease, arthritis and many types of cancer. This is proven by epidemiological studies of billions of people comparing cultures that eat a lot of red meat (e.g. all European nations) to ones that eat very little (e.g. most all Asian countries). Ideally, you would eat no meat at all, and you cannot eat meat if you are ill. You do not have to be a strict vegetarian to be healthy, but you cannot eat much meat at all regularly and stay well. If you choose to eat meat, eat small four-ounce portions of lean cuts that are low in fat no more than three times a week. If you cut the meat into small portions, marinate it and stir-fry it with vegetables Asian style it will go a lot further and you will enjoy it a lot more. Organically raised meat (poultry, eggs, milk or dairy) is still meat - don't kid yourself.

Poultry and eggs are also high in saturated fat, high in calories, low in fiber and have a very unbalanced nutrient profile. Poultry and eggs are also two of the top ten allergenic foods. You may be allergic to one or both, and not even be aware of it. There may be no overt and obvious symptoms right after eating them. You really should give up eggs completely. You should give up poultry as well although it is ubiquitous in our culture. No matter how organic or "free range" the poultry or eggs are, they are still poultry and eggs and contain large amounts of fat, cholesterol and

55

animal protein, and are no less allergenic. Eggs contain a whopping 250 mg of pure cholesterol each.

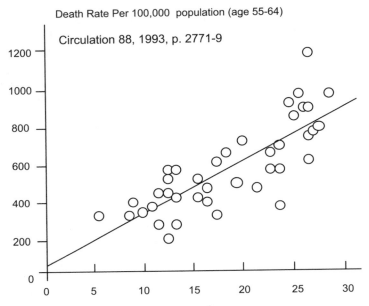

Death Rate Per 100,000 population (age 55-64)

Circulation 88, 1993, p. 2771-9

Cholesterol Saturated Fat Index per 1000 kcal/day
The more saturated fat you eat the more coronary
heart disease you get based on 40 countries.

Milk and dairy products are also high in saturated fats, high in calories, have no fiber and have a very unbalanced ratio of various vitamins and minerals. Most cultures do not drink milk or eat dairy products at all. Some people mistakenly assume that drinking low fat milk and eating low fat/ no fat dairy products is the answer. The problem is that all dairy products (except hard cheeses which are very high in saturated fat by nature) contain lactose or milk sugar. Lactose cannot be digested by any adult of any race since we lose the ability to produce the enzyme lactase at about the age of three. Africans and Asians are notoriously lactose intolerant, and Caucasians are just less obviously intolerant. Man is the only mammal that drinks milk after weaning. Yogurt, which is traditionally touted as a "health food" is worse because it contains twice the amount of lactose as regular milk.

Why? Because milk powder is added to yogurt to make it thicker. Stop drinking milk and stop using dairy products. Go to www.notmilk.com as well as www.milksucks.com to read more about the many reasons to take all dairy out of your life. Substitute with soy milk and meltable soy cheeses. There are also rice, oat and almond milks available, so keep trying them until you find one you really like. More and more you will see vegetarian replacements for dairy products like yogurt, sour cream, cream cheese and others. Buying expensive organic milk and dairy products is just deluding yourself - they are almost as bad as the regular ones. Many people have seen their health improve dramatically just by taking milk and dairy products out of their diets for a month.

Whole grains are literally the "staff of life" and should be the basis of your diet. Whole wheat, brown rice, corn, barley, buckwheat, rye, oats and millet are, and have been, the basis of human nutrition around the world for centuries basically. How many whole grains do you eat every day? Whole grains are low in fat, low in calories, have high quality protein, are full of fiber and have an excellent nutritional profile. They are also very non-allergenic; the repeated fallacies that wheat and corn are common allergens just aren't true. Allergies to any grain are rare, and brown rice may be the least allergenic of all foods. It is very easy to have brown rice or whole wheat pasta for dinner instead of white rice or white pasta. Chain grocery stores now carry 100% whole grain breads without preservatives. Discover polenta and corn bread. Make some barley soup. Cook up some buckwheat or millet one night and see how you like it. Have whole grain cold cereals or hot oatmeal for breakfast. Get creative with whole grains!

Beans are considered by some to be a food for poor people, but they are a staple of any healthy diet. There are many types of beans and you can find beans in Latin grocery stores you have never even heard of. Like whole grains, beans are low in fat, low in calories, have excellent protein, are loaded with fiber and have a good assortment of nutrients. Allergies to beans are rare and this includes supposed soybean allergies. The modern soybean has been bred to be high in oil content, but very few people eat cooked dried soybeans anyway.

Get a good recipe book and learn how to cook beans in various ways. You'll find they taste as good as they are good for you. Pinto, black, lentils, chickpeas, pink, kidney, adzuki, chili, black-eyed, limas, fava, navy, northern and cannelini are just some of the varieties you can find in stores.

Green and yellow vegetables are the next desirable food to eat, but not every one of them. Most vegetables are healthful and important for the nutrients like beta-carotene they contain. Vegetables have almost no fat, are very low in calories, contain lots of fiber and provide certain nutrients that only vegetables can provide like lignans and sterols. It is the Nightshade family that should be avoided; this includes potatoes, tomatoes, eggplants and peppers. Vegetables in the Nightshade family contain toxic alkaloids like solanine. If you extracted the solanine from a 100 pound bag of potatoes and ate it you would literally fall over dead. Potatoes, tomatoes, peppers and eggplants have dangerous and deleterious amounts of solanine in them and should only be eaten occasionally at most. For centuries tomatoes were considered an ornamental, toxic plant not fit for humans or animals to eat. In many cultures Nightshade plants such as tomatoes are not eaten at all. Learn to cook fresh vegetables in various international styles. Vegetables are very low in calories and fat. A good way to lose weight is to temporarily go on an all vegetable diet or an all vegetable soup diet for a week.

Fruits, surprisingly, are not very nutritious and should only be about 10% of your diet. Most all fruits are basically just sugar and water with very little nutrition and a very poor nutrient profile. Look at a nutritional analysis of any common fruit and you'll see it has almost no biologically significant amount of any vitamin or mineral whatsoever except for a little vitamin A or C. Dried fruits and fruit juices are even higher in sugar and should be avoided. A glass of fruit juice has as much sugar as a soft drink, and all simple sugars are basically the same. All sweeteners are harmful in excess. Whether the sugar is sucrose, dextrose, fructose or maltose it is still a simple sugar and should only be eaten in small amounts. Tropical fruits are meant for tropical people living in hot climates - like India. They are very allergenic, and citrus fruits, for example, are one of the top ten allergenic foods (lemons, limes, grapefruits, oranges and tangerines). Most vegetarians tend to be sugar addicts and eat large amounts of fruits, dried fruits, fruit juice, honey, maple syrup and other sweeteners. Thus, they have the same health problems as people who eat plain old white sugar. Sugar is sugar is sugar regardless of its source.

Seafood can be an important part of your diet if you don't want to be a vegetarian. A few people do have allergies to seafood, and these allergies may not be obvious. Fish and shellfish can be eaten in moderation regularly (i.e. a four ounce portion daily) if you choose to. I have never once seen any study to show that pure vegetarians are any healthier than those who add seafood to their diets. Choose low fat white fish like flounder, snapper and sole over high fat types such as catfish and turbot or fatty, dark skinned fish like swordfish, tuna and salmon which can contain 30% or more fat calories.

It should be mentioned there is no botanical category known as "nuts". Tree nuts such as almonds, walnuts, pecans, hazelnuts and others are unrelated botanically. They are very, very high in fat (over 70% generally), very high in calories, contain an unbalanced nutritional profile and should only be used in small amounts as garnish for your other foods. Peanuts are tropical legumes are not nuts at all. Peanuts are very allergenic and one of the top ten allergenic foods known. Give up nut butters altogether as they are so inordinately high in oil content.

You'll find that most of the popular diet authors are very uninformed and misleading - to put it politely. The most popular diet in history is the Atkins diet where you eat all the meat and fat you want, but avoid all complex carbohydrates like brown rice and whole grain bread. This is also called the "ketogenic" or Paleolithic diet and is based on the "glycemic index". Has anyone ever pointed out to you that "ketogenic" is based on a state of ketosis? Ketosis is defined as a pathological state of disease where you have excessive ketones in the body as in diabetes, acidosis and other conditions. Go look up "ketogenic" in your dictionary. The glycemic index is too silly to even talk about since they class simple carbohydrates as identical to complex carbohydrates. The glycemic index advocates irrationally claim brown rice is the same as white sugar, and a bowl of oatmeal is the same as a sugared donut! How can intelligent people even listen to this kind of thing?

Another fad diet is the one based on your blood type. Type O are Meat Eaters, type A are Vegetarians, type B are Nomads and type AB are Enigmas. This diet now has followers around the world who eat the wrong foods because they happen to have a certain blood type. Ladies, your blood type has almost no relevance at all except when you need a blood transfusion. This diet has people eating eggs, milk and dairy products, red meat and all kinds of unhealthy foods while telling them it is their biological destiny to eat this way!

Most all of the popular diet authors you see today have very poor advice for you on how to eat. In fact there are very few good authors out there who are sincere, practice what they preach and are good examples of what they advise. Dean Ornish is very good and is now a member of the Physician's Committee for Responsible Medicine. Neal Barnard is also a very sincere writer and member of the PCRM. You've probably seen Susan Powter on television and she writes excellent books like "Stop the Insanity", especially from a woman's perspective. Gary Null is a prolific writer who practices what he preaches and makes a lot of sense telling people that natural foods taste better than the refined ones most of us eat. Robert Pritikin followed in his father's tradition and has a very practical approach to eating well and staying slim. John McDougall writes books and publishes a newsletter. Terry Shintani wrote an excellent book called "The Hawaii Diet" on how to enjoy natural foods. If you have never read anything on the "macrobiotic" or Zen diet please read my "Zen Macrobiotics for Americans", especially if you are sick or have a chronic illness. This is the only book in the world to make the whole grain diet practical, varied, fun and delicious and take the unnecessary and restrictive Japanese influence out of it. There are many good books on traditional macrobiotics and Michio Kushi is probably the leading author, but please take out all the unnecessary Japanese trappings. People have literally cured cancer and other "incurable" illnesses by eating a whole grain based diet and written books like "My Beautiful Life", "Recalled By Life", "Recovery from Cancer" and "Confessions of a Kamikaze Cowboy" relating their healing with natural means instead of allopathic medicine.

Chapter 15: Losing Weight

Diets don't work...nobody wants to go hungry. If you eat whole natural healthy foods you can honestly eat all you want and lose weight. Do not even think of "going on a diet"- just make better food choices. It really is that simple...choose healthier natural foods. Will power is an illusion, and hunger is one of the strongest instincts we have, along with sexual desire - only hunger is by far the much stronger instinct. People can go years without sex, but only hours without food before complaining about hunger. Over half of Americans are medically overweight and more than 20% are clinically obese. You now see many overweight and obese children and teenagers. This entire situation has really only occurred in the last 30 years. Look at those TV shows from the early 1970's and see how most everyone is slim. What has happened in three decades? America is now the fattest nation on earth with the highest intake of fat calories. Don't think it is simply food that makes you fat; it is FAT that makes you fat. All those sugars and refined, nutritionless calories only make it worse.

You do not have to go hungry to lose weight. You couldn't do it if you wanted to anyway. Do you know one person who is able to go hungry and not eat for more than a few hours? The inherent desire to eat to stay alive is too instinctual and too ingrained in us. You just need to choose better foods to eat so you can eat whenever you are honestly hungry. What does "honestly hungry" mean? If you are honestly hungry you will be very happy to eat something simple like a piece of whole grain bread with apple butter on it, a bowl of hot or cold cereal, a piece of fruit or something else simple, natural and tasty. If you want, say, a piece of chocolate cake, you aren't really hungry but just looking for some emotional satisfaction. So, it is not a matter of how much you eat but WHAT you eat. Just make better food choices. You can actually eat more food every day and take in less calories by choosing whole grains, beans, vegetables, fruits, soups, salads and seafood, rather than meat, poultry, eggs, milk, dairy products, refined foods and sweetened foods.

The people in the countryside of Asia, for example, are generally poor and agrarian, but they have a surprisingly high calorie consumption. They cannot afford to eat red meat, poultry or eggs in any quantity, and dairy products are not a part of their culture. Therefore they exist mostly on grains such as rice, wheat and barley and lots of vegetables. They only eat about 15% fat calories, and these fat calories are mostly from vegetables and not animal foods. Obesity is uncommon, as are most forms of cancer, diabetes, heart/artery disease and other illnesses. Their food choices are largely forced on them by a lack of affluence, but they eat a lot and stay slim generally. This is basically true in countries like Indonesia, China, Thailand, Burma, Viet Nam, Korea and Japan. The city dwellers in countries like Japan more and more have adopted the Western diet and now eat more beef, pork, chicken, milk, cheese, yogurt, butter, eggs and other high calorie, high fat animal foods. As they do their health proportionately deteriorates and their disease rates more and more match those of the Western countries.

The popular fad diets simply don't work. There are count-less books on diet, and if one of these books worked there wouldn't be a problem anymore. The current fad in 2003 is still the "ketogenic" diet (discussed in the previous chapter), which doesn't work at all. There are no magic supplements that will make you lose weight either, although billions of dollars of diet aids are sold every year. There are no prescription drugs that will make you lose weight. You can take amphetamine based drugs temporarily to lose weight, but the psychological/mental/emotional side effects of regular and chronic amphetamine use are very severe. It is up to you to choose better foods to eat by reading books on natural health and educating yourself about what is best to eat. Making better food choices is not a "diet" at all, because you eat all you want and eat delicious natural foods. This is a matter of changing your lifestyle and being more aware of what you eat. You can honestly eat whenever you are hungry and maintain a normal weight for your height. Most of the diet books available are really awful and the authors don't have a clue as to the best foods to eat. Fortunately there are a few very sincere authors who do know what they are doing and do practice what they preach. A good example of this is Dean Ornish's book "Eat More, Weigh Less." Another fine example is Susan Powter's "Stop the Insanity." Any of the books by Gary Null, John McDougall, Neal Barnard, Robert Pritikin, Michio Kushi or Terry Shintani are very helpful. These authors suggest you eat whole grains, vegetables, fruits, salads, beans and even some seafood to lose weight and be healthy. Please be sure to read my "Zen Macrobiotics for Americans" - the only book ever written that makes the powerful macrobiotic diet practical, fun, tasty and varied. This is macrobiotics with all the unnecessary Japanese culture and influence taken out of it. Go to your local library and look up some of these authors and read what they have to say. It is not a matter of will power at all but, rather, of understanding what is best to eat. Diets don't work - you just need to make better food choices and you can actually eat all you want to eat and not gain weight.

A study was done at the University of Hawaii (American Journal of Clinical Nutrition vol. 53, 1991) by Dr. Shintani. Twenty obese Native Hawaiians in very poor health were put on their native high complex carbohydrate, moderate protein and low fat diet for only three weeks. THEY ATE ALL THEY WANTED! They ate taro, breadfruit, yams, green vegetables, local fruit, seafood and chicken (a half pound) as their ancestors did. In just 21 days they lost an average of over 17 pounds each, lowered their blood pressure, lowered their cholesterol and lowered their blood sugar all very dramatically with no exercise or supplements. This is real world proof that you can eat all you want and stay slim all your life if you'll just make better food choices. It is fat that makes you fat and not food that makes you fat.

At Cornell University in New York another human clinical study (American Journal of Clinical Nutrition vol. 46, 1987) proved you can eat all you want and stay slim as long as you choose low fat foods. These subjects were not even fed whole natural foods yet they lost weight on the low fat diet. Whole, natural foods would have obviously given even better results. Everyone was given the same foods, which only varied in the amount of fat calories. For example everyone got bran muffins but some were full of butter and eggs and others were not. Everyone ate all they wanted to without restriction. The ones on the low fat foods ate a mere 2,087 calories a day while the ones eating the high fat foods ate 2,714 calories. This was only a two week study but based on these results the healthy group would expect to lose 23 pounds a year while the unhealthy group would expect to gain 18 pounds a year.

At the University of Alabama another human study (American Journal of Clinical Nutrition vol. 37, 1983) was done to see how many calories people would eat given unrestricted access to foods varying in fat content. They were not weighed as the doctors only wanted to determine caloric intake. The ones who ate the low fat foods only averaged 1,570 calories a day even though they could eat all they wanted. The ones who ate the high fat foods averaged 3,000 calories which is almost twice as much.

One practice that will help is to eat a hot, hearty bowl of soup before lunch and before dinner each day. Eating hot, diluted soup makes us feel full and fulfills our hunger on far less calories. Eating soup at least once a day will lower your caloric intake significantly while completely satisfying your hunger. Get some soup cookbooks and get in the habit of having soup for lunch and dinner every day.

Your hormones can affect your weight very much and be responsible for some (emphasis on the word "some") of your excess pounds. An underactive thyroid gland can cause weight gain. You must test your T3 and T4 thyroid levels to see if they are normal. Overweight women have been shown to be universally low in estriol. You can easily and inexpensively do this with a saliva test kit since medical doctors never test for it. Estradiol and estrone are well known to often be high in overweight women. The only way to lower them is through total lifestyle and a low fat, high fiber diet, exercise, and limiting or avoiding alcohol. High insulin levels due to insulin resistance are very common in women over 40. Find a doctor who will give you a glucose tolerance test (GTT) to find out your insulin level. Please read Topic 13: Progesterone and Diabetes to learn how to normalize your blood sugar and insulin levels naturally. Be sure to test all your hormone levels and balance them as much as possible since our entire endocrine system works together harmoniously. Please see the chart of Basic Hormones at the back of the book to see the 16 vital hormones you should be concerned with.

Topic 16: Natural Arthritis Relief

Arthritis and joint inflammation affects at least 95% of Americans in old age. Interestingly enough this is not true in poorer countries where they can't afford to overeat and eat the wrong foods. Medical doctors have almost nothing to offer here, despite their constant claims to new "medical breakthroughs". Did you notice that none of their highly media acclaimed breakthroughs ever turn out? Again, they are trying to stamp out the symptom without addressing the cause. No matter how much advertising you see these wonder drugs never do work. The big push in 2003 is still "cox-2 inhibitors"- which don't work either.

Progesterone has been shown to be intimately related to arthritic conditions, but you are never told this. Over 60 years ago a study was published (Mayo Clinic Proceedings (1938) vol. 13, p. 161-7) about the relationship of progesterone levels in women and joint inflammation. This was first observed in pregnant arthritic women who often experienced great improvement as their progesterone levels went up during their pregnancy. In the Romanian journal Spitatul (1969, vol. 82, 1970, vol. 83 and 1971, vol. 84) studies were published showing progesterone balances or opposes the inflammatory nature of estrogens and is itself anti-inflammatory. Another study was done (Arthritis and Rheumatism (1986) vol. 29, p. 411-14) showing the relationship of progesterone levels to inflammation. The researchers found generally lower progesterone levels in women with arthritic conditions. Further studies in Japan on this were published in the Japanese Journal of Pharmacology in 1979. Yet another study (Journal of Rheumatism (1992) vol. 19, p. 1895-2000) showed that postmenopausal arthritic women were generally low in DHEA, androstenedione and progesterone compared to healthy women. Many women have reported lessening of their symptoms when using transdermal progesterone to treat their other problems. There are over a dozen published clinical studies showing the relationship between progesterone levels and joint inflammation. Since this can't be patented who will research this further?

The most important thing you can do for joint inflammation is to eat a low calorie, low sugar, high fiber, plant based, low fat, low protein, high complex carbohydrate diet of whole natural foods. A study (Drug Therapy Series (1992) vol. 5, p. 67-79) found a strong relationship between what people ate and how much arthritis they got. Much of this has to do with food allergies but, unfortunately, we do not have the technology to diagnose them. The ALCAT, ELISA and other such supposed allergy tests just don't work and are most inconsistent. Using food elimination techniques are almost impossible since many allergies are subtle, hidden or delayed in action. Many people have improved their conditions by taking Nightshade vegetables out of their diets. This includes potatoes, tomatoes, eggplants and peppers all of which contain toxic alkaloids like solanine. A study (American Medical News January 25, 1999, p. 45-7) recently proved the strong allergenic nature of Nightshade vegetables on hospital patients. Other studies (Journal of Clinical and Biological Chemistry (1996) vol. 20, p. 1-26) have shown that inflammation of the joints is largely dependent on what foods you eat. The worst foods you can eat to worsen inflammation are fats, especially saturated animal fats and hydrogenated oils (Pharmacology (1995) vol. 51, p. 160-4). The worst "food" you can eat are again the hydrogenated and partially hydrogenated oils (aka trans fatty acids), as they do not exist in nature and cause myriad problems (British Journal of Nutrition (1989) vol. 61, p. 519-29) such as clogged arteries, stroke, heart attack and altered hormone levels. People in poor countries that eat a healthier diet than us suffer from far less bone and joint problems (Nutrition Research (1994) vol. 14, p. 519-29), since they eat less calories, less meat, less sugar and less refined foods. Besides eating better food you can eat less food. Stop eating three unnecessary meals a day and start eating two meals every day. You can go even further and have a light snack in the morning or at noon and eat just one basic meal a day. The average woman only needs about 1,200 calories a day, and most women in America probably eat twice that much. The less you eat the longer you live and the healthier you are (Science, August 27, 1999). Fasting on water only can produce immediate and dramatic effects. Some excellent books on fasting have been written by Bueno, Cott, Adamson, Bragg and Fuhrman. Fasting is the most powerful healing technique known and can produce miracles.

What supplements can you take for arthritis? Our intestinal health has a strong influence on inflammation (Scandinavian Journal of Immunology (1994) vol. 40, p. 648-52) so you can take acidophilus, FOS and L-glutamine as discussed in the supplements chapter.

Glucosamine sulfate is good for arthritis, but must be supported by the right vitamins and all known minerals to be effective as it can't work alone. This is why some people get no relief from a glucosamine supplement used by itself. Boswellin extract is another proven supplement that comes from India and is commonly available when 250 mg (10% boswellic acids) of a reliable brand is taken. Flax oil - one or two grams a day - is very good, and a better choice than fish liver oils for a variety of reasons. MSM or methyl sulfonyl methane is, in a way, an oral form of DMSO that has been promoted. After all these years there is not one published clinical study showing its value however. Curcumin is an extract of turmeric and is a very powerful antioxidant. Take 500 mg of actual curcumin in your supplement for a variety of reasons and not just your arthritis. Curcumin is a very strong anti-inflammatory, lowers cholesterol and has anti-cancer properties. Plain gelatin is also known as hydrolyzed collagen and is a basic building block of cartilage. A popular name brand of this is available but rather overpriced. Take one to two tablespoons a day. Quercitin 250 mg is a powerful, effective and safe natural anti-inflammatory. Finally some studies have appeared on SAMe if you take enough of it (200 mg actual ionic SAMe).

There are four vitamins that have an established connection to inflammation and they are vitamins C, D, E and K. These are discussed in the supplement chapter. 250 mg of vitamin C is good, 800 IU of vitamin D, 400 IU of vitamin E (mixed tocopherols) and 80 or more mcg of vitamin K is suggested.

All thirteen of our basic known minerals are vital to healing inflammation, which includes calcium, magnesium, boron, copper, manganese, molybdenum, selenium, silica, chromium, iron, iodine, vanadium and zinc. Phosphorous, sulfur, potassium and sodium are plentiful in our diets. Search the Internet under "minerals" or "mineral supplements" to find one with all 13 in the formula in the amounts you need, as nearly all brands are inadequate. We may also need germanium, tin, nickel, strontium and cobalt.

Let's talk about what doesn't work and is merely a promotion of one type or another. Please understand that the chondroitin you see sold and advertised everywhere is worthless. Chondroitin is a molecule that is too large to pass through your intestinal wall and simply cannot be absorbed. It works only if a surgeon injects it directly into your joint. SOD (superoxide dismutase) will also work if injected directly into your joint, but not if you eat it. Ignore the advertising and do not waste any money on chondroitin; the "studies" are paid advertisements. CMO or cetyl myristoleate has been around for decades, but even its inventor (and only supporter) admits you need about 14 grams a day – and even that much wouldn't work. Ginger or ginger oil is another promotion without value for inflammation. Devils Claw is an African herb that has been known about for many years, but no one has been getting any relief from it in all this time. All these things are still actively being promoted though. Avoid them all.

Now let's talk about the other hormones that affect arthritis. DHEA, melatonin, pregnenolone and testosterone should be mentioned. DHEA falls as we have seen after the age of 20 generally. DHEA is vital for joint health (Arthritis and Rheumatism (1997) vol. 40, p. 907-11). You must have your blood or saliva measured so you'll know if you need to supplement this. Melatonin has been proven to be vital in joint health and inflammation. Your doctor doesn't know this nor care, since it is available without prescription. Studies (Zhonngua Yaolixue Tongbao (1994) vol. 10, p. 290-3) verify this, but even natural health researchers are unaware of this. Pregnenolone falls sharply after the age of 35 and is certainly involved with joint health, although we have no specific studies showing this. Remember that pregnenolone is the "forgotten" or orphan hormone and that all our hormones work together synergistically in concert supporting and helping each other. There are no studies I could find specifically on testosterone either, but we do know how important it is for bone health. Bone health and joint inflammation are almost identical in cause and treatment so it is necessary to measure your testosterone level with blood or saliva and see if you need supplementation.

Topic 17: Natural Supplements

There are many natural, safe, proven, effective and inexpensive supplements you can take to be healthier, have stronger immunity, feel better and live longer. Nothing will replace a good diet, however, so please don't think taking supplements will make up for not eating well. It is very confusing to choose which supplements to take, as nearly all of what you read is advertising promotion, rather than science, no matter how well written and which well compensated doctor is pushing it. The natural supplement industry is as bad as any other, sorry to say, and the real motivation for most of these people is profit rather than helping to make people healthier without drugs. There are a few good advocates out there though, and there are a few good companies. The following list of suggested supplements may sound like a very long one, but all of them will help you live a better and healthier life, avoid illness, live longer and avoid taking prescription drugs and getting surgery.

- A good multivitamin and mineral supplement is basic and will probably contain all the vitamins you need, but not all the minerals. Nearly all vitamins by necessity are synthesized despite claims to the contrary. It is better to buy a vitamins-only formula and take your minerals separately.
- Good mineral supplements are all but impossible to find with all 13 needed minerals - calcium, magnesium, iron 18 mg, selenium 70 mcg, chromium 120 mcg, boron 3 mg, copper 5 mg, silicon 10 mg, iodine 150 mcg, molybdenum 75 mcg, zinc 15 mg, manganese 2 mg and vanadium 1 mg. Search the Internet under "mineral supplements".
- Vitamin E 400 IU natural mixed tocopherols - the mixed tocopherols are the most natural and complete form.
- Vitamin B-6 only 10 mg. The RDA is 2 mg so this is 500% of what you need. Yes, some short term studies call for 50 mg or even more, but megadoses of any nutrient are contraindicated, even water soluble vitamins like this.

- NAC or N-acetyl cysteine 600 mg. This is a much better way to raise you glutathione (a basic antioxidant enzyme) levels than using glutathione itself.
- PS or phosphatidyl serine 100 mg. This is very important for brain function, and large amounts of PS are found in our brain tissue. Many good studies on this.
- Lecithin is an extract of soybeans and helps lower cholesterol and support good brain metabolism. A 1,200 mg softgel is good.
- Vitamin C only 250 mg. That's right - it's 400% of your RDA and you don't need any more than that. People who tell you to take megadoses of this or any other nutrient are misinformed quacks. Taking grams of vitamin C will acidify your blood and cause serious side effects over time.
- Beta Carotene 10,000 IU to 25,000 IU instead of vitamin A. This is a very basic and important antioxidant.
- Folic acid 400 to 800 mcg. Like vitamin B-6 this seems to have an important effect especially on women.
- Beta Sitosterol is an extract of sugar cane pulp. This is good for breast and uterine health, and will lower your cholesterol levels very effectively. You must use 300 mg to get good effects so read the label for contents.
- FOS (aka inulin) or fructooligosaccharides one or two 750 mg capsules a day to improve your intestinal flora. FOS is an indigestible sugar that feeds the good colon bacteria.
- Lactospore is the stable spore form of acidophilus that does not need refrigeration. Good with regular acidophilus.
- Aloe Vera taken orally is good for digestion, ulcers, blood sugar regulation and immunity. Use for 6-12 months only.
- Acidophilus 3 billion units a day. Buy it and keep it refrigerated. Buy only reputable, name brands that state "3 billion units per capsule" on the label. This will help keep your intestines flourishing with beneficial bacteria.
- Lipoic acid 200 mg to help keep blood sugar levels normalized. Lots of published science on this.
- Flax oil one or two 1,000 mg capsules a day. Buy this and keep this refrigerated. A one gram capsule is a mere 9 fat calories. This is the best known source of omega-3 fatty acids and better than fish oil.

- Chondroitin is not orally absorbed and must be injected directly into your joints to be effective. Do not fall for the advertising on this, as it simply cannot pass through our intestinal walls intact. This will just not help your arthritis.
- Glucosamine is a fine supplement for arthritis and joint inflammation in 500 mg or more doses. You need to take all thirteen known minerals to go with it for effectiveness as glucosamine needs co-factors in order to work.
- Vitamin D may already be in your multivitamin but only 400 IU. 800 IU is recommended. This is basically not found in any food you eat.
- Vitamin K 80 mcg is a very important vitamin and may be in your multivitamin. Vitamin K is the" forgotten vitamin" but is very important in our diets.
- Soy Isoflavones 40 mg are essential as you just aren't going to eat enough soy foods to get this amount. Do not listen to the anti-soy hysteria you may hear, as the studies on this run into the thousands. There is no reason to take more than 40 mg of genestein and diadzein.
- Magnesium about 200 to 400 mg of any type or brand you want. This is a vital mineral to take even if you are eating well. Calcium cannot be absorbed without sufficient magnesium as well as boron and vitamin D. This should be in your mineral supplement.
- Calcium about 400 to 800 mg (about twice the amount of magnesium you are taking). Citrate, carbonate, and other forms all absorb well. This should also be in your mineral supplement.
- L-glutamine one gram twice a day will do wonders for your intestines. It is inexpensive and has much science behind it. This will actually temporarily spike your levels of human growth hormone. A very important amino acid to take.
- Beta Glucan is the most potent immune system enhancer known to science. Taking 200 mg from either yeast or oats is the most important thing you can do to make your immunity stronger and resist illnesses and infections. The studies on this are overwhelming. Please read my book "What Is Beta Glucan?" This is a basic supplement.
- I3C or indole-3-carbinol is a vegetable extract from cabbage and other cruciferous vegetables. It is better to take its direct metabolite DIM (di-indolyl methane). This

71

proven supplement will improve estrogen metabolism and lower estrogen levels. Take no less than 200 mg of DIM as nearly all brands offer much less than this.

- CoQ10 or coenzyme Q 10 is a powerful antioxidant and vital for any good supplement program. You must take at least 100 mg to get real effects, and 200 mg if elderly or ill. CoQ10 has many proven benefits including anti-cancer activity and more studies are done on this all the time.
- Vitamin B-12 is important as we age, but is very, very poorly absorbed orally. Take 1,000 mcg of regular or sublingual. A nasal spray would be very effective, but is considered a "drug" by the FDA and cannot be sold without a prescription. Consider 10 mg of methyl cobalamin as it is claimed to be an orally available form of B-12.
- Curcumin is an extract of tumeric. Make sure this contains 400 to 500 mg of actual curcumoids per tablet listed on the label. Do not buy plain tumeric powder. This is a very powerful antioxidant, and anti-inflammatory that lowers cholesterol and has potent anti-cancer properties. Take only for one year as it is exogenous (not in regular food).
- Quercitin is a potent plant antioxidant that is not well known yet. More value for this is being found in women and you can take 250 to 500 mg of any good brand. There are good studies on this, it is not expensive and has strong benefits.
- Green Tea has potent polyphenols with many proven health benefits. Find a brand that is decaffeinated. Green tea even has proven anti-cancer activity.
- Acetyl-L-carnitine is good for brain metabolism and 500 mg is a good dose. Lots of good studies on this one to maintain good cognition into old age.
- Ellagic acid 100 mg or more is a good anti-cancer supplement but only for one year.
- Coral calcium, chondroitin, colloidal minerals, noni juice, ocean silver, deer antler velvet, maca root, colostrum, breast enhancers, OTC growth hormone supplements, colloidal silver, libido enhancers, lycopene, chorella, spirulina, homeopathic remedies and other such products are all overpriced promotions without any value.

Topic 18: Natural Hormone Balance

Why is it that medical doctors almost never test your hormone levels? Why in the world would they give a woman estrogen supplements without testing her levels of estradiol, estrone and estriol? And why don't doctors even know about estriol? Why are they almost completely disinterested in such vital, basic and important hormones as progesterone, DHEA, melatonin, testosterone, androstenedione, pregnenolone, cortisol, thyroid and growth hormone? Our hormone levels are critical in countless ways and central to our health, yet almost no one has any idea at all what their hormone profile looks like. We have already covered the three basic human estrogens and progesterone, so let's look at eight more of our most basic hormones.

DHEA is called the "life extension" hormone with good reason. As you can see by the chart DHEA levels fall after the age of 20 in both men and women, and are generally extremely low by the age of 60. However, it is possible to have too much as well as too little DHEA, so testing your levels is required. Having too high a level is just as harmful as having too little. If your level is too high it is only possible to lower it by diet, exercise and lifestyle. Unfortunately there are no known supplements that will help lower it. Ideally you should strive for the youthful level you enjoyed at about the age of 30. You can do this by taking 10-25 mg a day orally and monitoring your results after about three months, until you maintain where you want to be. Some women will need even higher doses especially if they are very old or ill. Several good books have been written on the importance of this hormone in how long we live, our immunity, menopause, sexual functioning and fulfillment, obesity, cholesterol, arthritis, cancers of many types, memory, high blood pressure, diabetes, stress, infections, sense of well being and sexual desire and fulfillment. Do not take this without testing to verify that your levels are low, as it is a very powerful and effective hormone that must be used intelligently.

Melatonin is secreted by the pineal gland and is called the "aging clock" hormone. Like DHEA this, in part, determines how

73

long we live. As you can see by the chart melatonin peaks when we are teenagers and declines through life until it all but disappears before we die. Anyone over 40 should be able to take about 3 mg of melatonin nightly. You can only take it at night as melatonin falls during the day when we perceive light and rises in the evening especially when we sleep. You must saliva test individually for this at 3:00 AM in the morning to monitor your levels. You can do this after about three months of supple- mentation. Melatonin is very underestimated currently, but clinical studies are showing just how vitally important it is for our health and longevity. Melatonin affects every cell in our body and has even shown anti-cancer activity in human studies. Several good books have been written on it, but even they can underestimate the power of this basic hormone. You will hear much more on this in the future.

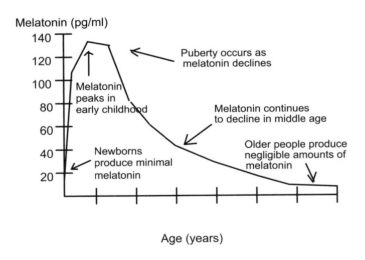

Age (years)

Why are we talking about *testosterone* for women? You only have about one tenth as much as men do, but testosterone is critical for many of your biological processes especially the building, maintenance and repair of your bones. Here you can also have too much as well as too little, and testing for testosterone levels is required. Like DHEA, this is important for sexual desire and fulfillment. If low you can see a doctor and get, say, a 0.3% natural testosterone cream or gel and monitor your

74

levels after, say, three months of use to make sure your dosage is correct. It is important to NEVER take oral testosterone salts or injections. You must use the natural cream or gel that is bio-identical. You are looking for a youthful level as you enjoyed around the age of 30. Men can use oral doses of androstenedione to raise their testosterone, but women should not because they metabolize this differently. So far no studies have been done on women using androstenedione. You can also test for andro-stenedione itself - it is also an important hormone for women, but usually parallels testosterone levels. Excessive levels of androstenedione cause health problems in women.

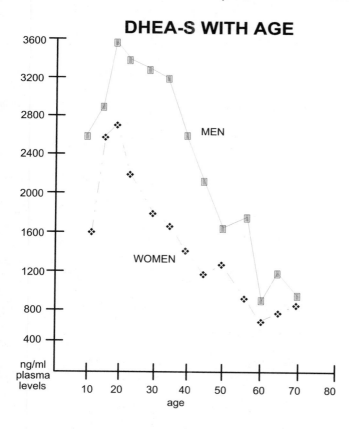

You have probably never even heard of **pregnenolone** as it is the "forgotten" or orphan hormone. It is pathetic that this basic hormone has so few studies available and so little research.

Pregnenolone is the precursor to all the other sex hormones and is therefore known as the "grandmother" of hormones. Medical doctors have no idea about its importance. As you can see by the chart your levels fall at about the age of 35 and then stabilize. This is THE most powerful memory enhancer known to science and the most important hormone for brain metabolism, yet we hardly know anything about it. If you study the published medical literature of the world you will find very few studies every year. A blood test can be specially ordered for about $150, but it is easier and less expensive to do saliva testing. If you are over 40 you can choose to take 25 mg a day about 5 days per week (men can usually take 50 mg daily) and then test yourself after three months. Again, you are looking for the youthful level you had at about age 30. To keep your brain healthy with a sharp mind and good memory pregnenolone supplementation is very important.

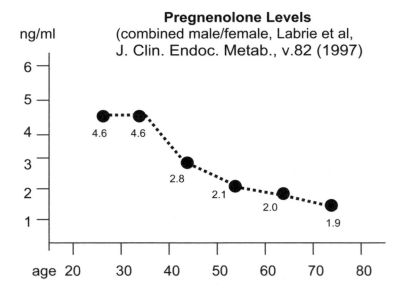

Pregnenolone Levels
(combined male/female, Labrie et al,
J. Clin. Endoc. Metab., v.82 (1997)

Growth hormone falls as we age and can only be measured by a blood test. You cannot use IGF-1 levels as an indicator regardless of the "conventional wisdom". Soon we will have saliva testing for this as well. Do not fall for the popular myth that IGF-1 levels (which can easily be saliva tested) accurately parallel GH levels, because this just isn't true. NONE of the supplements sold that promise to raise growth hormone work no matter how convincing the advertising. None of them! Do not buy any of these no matter how good they sound, because they don't work. Trust me on this, ladies. You can temporarily spike your growth hormone by taking one gram of the amino acid L-glutamine twice a day as mentioned in the supplement chapter, but this does not raise the level all day. Eating less, exercising, fasting, and not having bad habits like smoking all help keep growth hormone levels higher.

The only way to raise your levels is expensive injections of recombinant (synthesized) rhGH that will cost you about $300 to $500 a month. All OTC growth hormone supplements are useless scams and none of them work! If you can afford this cost and have proven your levels are low (or simply not youthful) you can inject this three times a week. Nasal spray secretagogues like hexarelin are safe and effective for humans, but will be just as expensive and are not currently approved for use in any country. Within ten years we will have less expensive (but not inexpensive) nasal sprays to safely and effectively raise our growth hormone levels. You may have heard unrealistic stories of "miraculous" benefits of taking growth hormone injections. Yes, you will get some positive benefits if you are, in fact, low in GH, but you must also balance all your other basic hormones to get the full value from this. Always remember that hormones work together as a harmonious team and support each other. Balance all of them.

We must mention *cortisol* or the stress hormone. Test this to see how you are doing. High levels indicate stress and low levels indicate longer life and better health. The only way to lower high cortisol levels is diet, lifestyle and dealing with whatever stress is causing the problem. Deficient cortisol levels are not usually found. There is reason to believe that a high DHEA to cortisol (i.e. high DHEA and low cortisol) ratio indicates longevity while a low DHEA to cortisol ratio indicates shorter life and weaker health.

Our thyroid gland is not well understood even with all the great medical advances that have been made. You must test your *T3* (2,3,5-triiodothyronine) and *T4* (L-thyroxine) separately and then supplement with bio-identical hormones if you are deficient.

77

You can also test your blood sugar and take a glucose tolerance test (GTT) to get an idea of the status of your blood sugar and insulin. Insulin is secreted by the pancreas, but is also influenced by the thyroid hormones. Insulin resistance happens when excess insulin is produced because it isn't accepted by the cells. This is a major problem in Western society and due in part to our extreme intake of various sugars. The prescription T3 (Cytomel) and T4 (Synthroid) hormones available at pharmacies are bio-identical fortunately. Some people choose to take animal gland extracts (Armour Thyroid) standardized for their T3 and T4 content in a 4:1 ratio, but this gives you both whether you need them or not. Test and take any needed thyroid hormones separately.

The *thymus* gland atrophies as we age. The thymus does not simply produce one hormone we can replace. The only thing you can do is take a good brand of a bovine dessicated thymus powder 500 to 1,000 mg a day.

You will surely find that whatever doctor you go to - medical or naturopathic - is very unfamiliar with your hormones, their effects, testing them and giving you proper supplements to correct any imbalances. Even expensive life extension clinics are generally incompetent in the area of natural hormone balance. Basically you are going to have to do this yourself and not depend on a medical professional of any kind. Fortunately, you have saliva testing available as well as reasonably priced blood testing. America is the only industrialized country in the world where you can legally buy most hormones over the counter inexpensively. This may stop at any time unfortunately and a prescription for, say, melatonin will end up costing you over $100 with a doctors visit and a prescription, rather than just $5 at the drugstore. Always remember that all our hormones act in concert and work together as a biological team. Don't just test and balance one or two hormones. Do your best to test all your basic hormones (see the list at the back of the book) and take the ones you need (and lower the ones that are excessive) to lead a long and healthy life. As we learn more and more about the importance and benefits of our endocrine systems and the hormones produced, the more doctors will be forced to routinely test your hormone levels. You are never going to be healthy and feel good if any of your hormones are out of balance.

Topic 19: Don't Get a Hysterectomy

It is simply inexcusable and criminal that one third of American women will end up being castrated by unnecessary hysterectomies. This is not something that happens just to elderly women - it generally occurs at an average age of about 40. Castrating a woman by removing her uterus is simply a barbaric act of unjustified butchery, except possibly for extreme cases such as advanced cancer. In poor, agrarian countries only about 1% of women undergo this radical operation. Over 600,000 hysterectomies are performed in the United States every year and most all of them completely unnecessary. Why do women slavishly and unquestioningly agree to this?

Men would never agree to have their testicles cut off. In fact, if doctors tried to castrate one third of all men - like they currently castrate women - they would be found hanging from telephone poles. If women were more educated about this the rate would fall to almost nothing. Most doctors will try to tell you the uterus and ovaries are "optional" organs that you only need until you're forty years old and don't want any more children. Please remember that when you get a hysterectomy your ovaries always atrophy and die. Doctors often purposely mislead women by telling them their ovaries will remain intact, while knowing full well they will not live due to lack of blood supply - your ovaries ALWAYS die after a hysterectomy. The side effects from losing your uterus and ovaries are played down and denied by doctors, but are extremely injurous and debilitating. Depression, mental disturbance and psychological problems from no longer having all their reproductive organs are universal and permanent. Most women feel they are no longer "intact" or "complete women" any more. The many other severe side effects include complete hormonal imbalance, urinary dysfunction, chronic fatigue, joint pain, bone loss, loss of libido, inability to enjoy sex and greatly increased rates of coronary heart disease and heart attacks and other disease conditions.

The main justifications given for this unnecessary and cruel procedure are pelvic infections, fibroids, endometriosis, bleeding and prolapse. Ladies, none of these common complaints justify such radical butchery and biological devastation. We've just discussed that fibroids and endometriosis are generally caused by excessive estrogen levels, and can be remedied naturally with changes in diet and lifestyle. Infection and bleeding can also be treated naturally without resorting to such an extreme procedure. Prolapse can be corrected by a specialist in gynecological surgery instead of removing the uterus.

What if you have already had this done? Fortunately, there is good news for you. Have your doctor give you a complete hormone scan of all your basic hormones or preferably saliva test them yourself. This would include DHEA, pregnenolone, testosterone, progesterone, estriol, estrone, estradiol, T3, T4, growth hormone and melatonin. Any that are low can easily be raised with supplementation. Any that are too high can be lowered with changes in diet and lifestyle. You can do a much better job of this at far less cost than doctors can. Your hormone profile can actually be better than the majority of women who have not undergone surgery since they have never tested and balanced their hormone levels. You would also want to make important changes in the food you eat, take all of the supplements recommended in Topic 17, get regular exercise and limit any bad habits. You can overcome the very serious side effects of this operation and live a long, healthy life in spite of it.

If your doctor has suggested a hysterectomy please find a new doctor. You don't need a doctor that wants to butcher you without just cause. Educate yourself by reading up on this and you'll surely come to see this is completely unnecessary in nearly every case. There are five very important books you should read on this subject, and four of them were written by women:

No More Hysterectomies, Vicki Hufnagel
How to Avoid a Hysterectomy, Lynn Payer
The Hysterectomy Hoax, Stanley West
The Castrated Woman, Naomi Stokes
Hysterectomy Before & After, Winnifred Cutler

Topic 20: Various Benefits of Progesterone

This is a catchall chapter in no particular order where some of the many and varied scientifically documented benefits of progesterone supplementation will be discussed. Natural progesterone cannot be patented, so there is little incentive to keep studying the many wonderful potential uses. We've already seen how valuable it is, and we'll see even more value in the future.

Progesterone is highly concentrated in the brain and is integral to brain function and cognition. Progesterone is second only to pregnenolone in brain metabolism. Progesterone protects our brains from stroke and helps repair damage after injury or trauma. Studies on this have been published in Brain Research 1993 and 1996, Experimental Neurology 1994 and other journals.

Progesterone is beneficial when treating atherosclerosis, which is the buildup of plaque in our arteries. It helps to normalize cholesterol and triglyceride levels in test animals. Such studies were published in Journal of Drug Research 1974 and Atherosclerosis 1996. Other blood irregularities such as high uric acid levels are common as we age. At the Eliada Hospital in Athens it was found progesterone lowered uric acid levels with no change in diet. Dietary changes are usually the only safe and effective way to do this.

At Stanford University in California test animals were more sexually active when given progesterone as opposed to those that were given estrogen supplements. This was published in Hormones and Behavior in 1980. Progesterone is erotic.

Progesterone helps us to adapt to and deal with stress more effectively. Stress more than anything else is responsible for the epidemic of high blood pressure in industrialized countries. Stress is more damaging to our health than poor diet or lack of exercise. A good study on this was published in Brain Research in 1995. Blood pressure tends to be raised by estradiol but reduced by progesterone. At the University of Pennsylvania doctors demonstrated this as well as other negative effects of excess estradiol on women's blood lipids. Oral contraceptives with their unnatural estrogens are known to adversely affect blood pressure. More studies were done on progesterone and blood pressure at Queen's University in Belfast, at McMaster University in Ontario and the University of Kumaoto in Japan. These studies were published in the Japan Heart Journal 1978, Hypertension Physiology Treatment 1977, Microcirculation 1st 1976, Kardiologiya 1977, and Artery 1980.

In Psychoneuroendocrinology 1992 women were found to have better memories during the luteal phase of their periods when progesterone levels are the highest. This becomes more important as women age and their levels fall. Senility, memory loss and Alzheimer's are due in part to low progesterone levels.

Remember that the word "progesterone" comes for PROGESTation as it promotes fertility and conception. Progest-erone helps to prevent natural and spontaneous abortions even when toxic abortive chemicals are injected into test animals. Studies were published in Nippon Juishikai Zasshi 1989 and Shengzhi Yu Biyun 1989 verifying these effects.

Many women, even in their twenties and thirties, have anovulatory periods where they produce no progesterone as no eggs are released from either ovary. There is no practical and effective way to know this is occurring. Such women have high rates of amenorrhea and other menstrual problems. Progesterone deficiency in amenorrhea was established in Chinese studies and published in Shanxi Yixue Zazhi 1988. Edema or water retention is a common menstrual complaint. Studies at a major Moscow Hospital found edema could be reduced with progesterone supplementation as it lowered excessive aldosterone levels. Dysmenorrhea with heavy bleeding is another common complaint. At the Los Olivos Medical Clinic in California this was successfully treated with progesterone and the results published in the Journal of Reproductive Medicine 1978. Dysmenorrhea, or problematic periods, is known to be generally caused by estrogen dominance, especially estradiol. Obviously progesterone supplementation is a major therapy to remedy this. The British Journal of Obstetrics and Gynecology 1979 published a study to demonstrate the effectiveness of this. At the University of Iowa it was established that many menstrual disorders are due to low progesterone levels. This can lead to infertility and impaired ability to conceive as reported in the Journal of Clinical Endocrinology and Metabolism 1974.

Progesterone affects all the other endocrine glands and hormone levels and is critical to their proper function. When progesterone levels are low the other hormones cannot work at their optimal efficiency. One example is that progesterone stimulates the parathyroid gland to produce higher PTH levels. This was shown in Journal of Clinical Endocrinology and Metabolism 1988.

Progesterone has the ability to help kill dangerous microorganisms such as the deadly orthopox virus. The antiviral power of progesterone was reported in the Journal of Veterinary Medical Service B, 1987. In Glasgow doctors showed how progesterone strengthens our immunity by improving leukocyte function and published their findings in Immunological Factors in Humans 1983. Herpes simplex has been an epidemic for decades now with almost no medical means to control it. Doctors at Pennsylvania State University found they could kill 87% of herpes virus in test cultures simply by adding an extremely weak solution of progesterone. Further studies in humans are needed here.

Epilepsy is an all too common electrical brain disorder that is in part hormonally caused. Progesterone is so heavily concentrated in the brain it is very rational to see that normal progesterone levels are needed in order to treat people with epilepsy. At the University of Umea in Sweden this was clearly demonstrated and published in Acta Physiologica Scandinavia 1987. Why aren't doctors using progesterone for their epileptic patients instead of numbing their brains with drugs?

That progesterone can help heal gastric ulcers is also unknown to the medical profession. This was demonstrated at the Medical College in Miraj, India and also at the University of Nigeria. These studies were published in the Indian Journal of

Medical Research 1977 and Journal of Pharmacology 1984. Natural therapies like this are far more effective than drugs.

The epidemic of anorexia, bulimia and other eating disorders is a very recent development in Western society, yet is almost unknown in Third World countries. Anorexia nervosa was studied at the Endocrinological Clinic in Warsaw. The doctors there found a clear tendency towards high estrogen levels and low progesterone levels in women with various eating disorders. This study was published in Acta Endocrinologica 1979.

Better sleep may well come with using progesterone according to Japanese researchers at Saitama Medical College. See Kagaku to Seibutsu 1979. Doesn't this sound like a more promising therapy than sleeping pills that cause mental and emotional side effects?

It has been well established that men can also benefit from progesterone supplementation. Progesterone is not a feminine hormone, but rather a human hormone, and men merely have lower levels of this than women. After the age of 50 men generally have higher levels of estradiol and estrone than their postmenopausal wives do! That's right, after 50 estrogen falls in women but rises in men. This is a very negative endocrinological situation and causes a variety of conditions. This is especially true with prostate enlargement and prostate cancer, which are epidemics in western societies. Prostate cancer is the leading cause of cancer in Western men and is caused in large part by estrogen dominance. The men in your life can also benefit from using small (1/8th teaspoon) amounts of transdermal progesterone cream directly on their scrotum five days a week. Please have them read my book, "The Natural Prostate Cure" for research on this and other natural therapies.

When using natural progesterone over a long period of time you may well find that certain conditions and problems you have lived with for years just plain disappear. Problems you had just given up on and accepted as an inevitable part of aging may just go away since your immune system will be stronger, your hormones will be more in balance, and your entire body metabolism will be improved.

Topic 21: Home Hormone Testing

It is very important you test the levels of your basic hormones that we have discussed. You can go to a doctor and get blood tests done but these are invasive, expensive, require an office visit, and blood must be drawn. Doctors are very uneducated about hormones generally and don't even know the difference between bound (not bio-available) and unbound (bio-available) levels. Words like "melatonin", "progesterone", "DHEA", "estriol" and "pregnenolone", just aren't in their vocabulary. Often doctors will actually call unnatural, synthetic progestins "progesterone" and mislead you to believe that is what you're getting. Proteins in our blood (called sex hormone binding globulins or SHBG) attach themselves to most of our sex hormones and make them biologically unavailable. About 98% of testosterone, for example, is bound and unavailable yet the doctors will often check that as if it has any meaning. DHEA can be tested free or as DHEA-S, which is the sulfate form.

Fortunately, there is another way to do this at home easily and inexpensively by buying a saliva hormone test kit. Saliva testing for hormones has been done in clinics for decades, but was never available to individual doctors much less consumers. Bringing this to the retail market inexpensively is one of the greatest technological medical breakthroughs of the decade. Now anyone can test their basic hormones for about $30 without a doctor. The World Health Organization approved this in the early 1990's for its ease, efficiency and practicality especially in the field where refrigeration was not available. You simply purchase a kit, which contains a plastic tube, and mail a sample of your saliva to the lab. They analyze this with sophisticated RIA (radioimmuno assay) apparatus and send you the results. You also get a chart to compare your levels according to sex and age.

Generally these labs test basic hormones for about $30 each although the price varies somewhat. Search the Internet under "saliva hormone tests" to find sources. Melatonin has to be ordered separately and tested at 3:00 AM in the morning. Vegetarians and people who eat seafood (but no meat or dairy) will generally have lower levels of sex hormones (cortisol and melatonin are not sex hormones). Always test your levels at the same time each morning, say, 8:00 AM, and do not brush your teeth beforehand or the results will not be valid. Estradiol, estrone, estriol and progesterone must be tested at exact times of your period if you are premenopausal as they vary greatly during the month.

Here are five labs, which are the main ones in the U.S. currently offering this service:

Aeron Life Cycle Labs
(now sold thru Jason Products)
8469 Warner Drive
Culver City, CA   90232
(800) 527-6605 toll free

Great Smokies Diagnostics
(aka Body Balance)
18-A Regent Park Blvd.
Asheville, NC   28806
(888) 891-3061 toll free

ZRT Labs
1815 N.W, 169th Place #3090
Beaverton, OR   97006
(503) 466-2445 phone
www.salivatest.com

Pharmasan
375 280th Street
Osceola, WI   54020
(888) 342-7272)
www.pharmasan.com

Life-Flo Health Care Products
11202 North 24th Avenue
Phoenix, AZ   85029
(888) 999-7440
www.life-flo.com

Books to Read

Not all the following books are great, by any means, but they all have something valuable to offer. If you don't see a prominent author mentioned here it is probably because they are still promoting the "value" of estrogen replacement and progestins and the supposed "benefits" of HRT generally. You'll still find some unsound and misleading advice in many of these books and some of the authors are still taken in by some of the many estrogen myths.

I would love to expose some of the really bad books for women - especially those by the most popular, but very misguided and uninformed authors. It is considered "bad form" in the publishing business to do this, however, so there is no list of "Books Not to Read".

PMS- A Guide- Katharina Dalton
Once a Month- Katharina Dalton
Natural Progesterone for Women- John Lee
What Your Doctor May Not Tell You About Menopause- John Lee
What Your Doctor May Not Tell You About Premenopause- John Lee
The Estrogen Alternative- Raquel Martin
Natural Woman, Natural Menopause- Marcus Laux
Hormone Heresy- Sherrill Sellman
Natural Progesterone- Anna Rushton
Natural Hormone Replacement- Jonathan Wright
Holistic Menopause- Judy Hall
Menopause without Medicines- Linda Ojeda
Menopausal Years- Susun Weed
The Menopause Industry- Susan Coney
For Women Only- Gary Null (any books by Gary)
Natural Treatments for Menopause- The Natural Pharmacist
O.K., So, I Don't Have a Headache- Christine Ferrare
Menopause- Michael Murray
Menopause- Edna Ryneveld

Natural Choices for Menopause- Marilyn Glenville
The HRT Solution- Marla Ahlgrimm
Eat More, Weigh Less- Dean Ornish (anything by Dean)
McDougall Program for Women- John McDougall (anything by John)
Stop the Insanity!- Susan Powter (anything by Susan)
The Pritikin Principle- Robert Pritikin (anything by Robert)
Dr. Shintani's Hawaii Diet- Terry Shintani
Save Yourself from Breast Cancer- Robert Kradjian
My Beautiful Life- Milenka Dobic
What's Your Menopause Type?- Joseph Collins
The Menopause Manager- Mary Mayo
Perimenopause the Natural Way- Eldred Taylor
Get Off the Menopause Roller Coaster- Shari Lieberman
Wisdom of Menopause- Christiane Northup
It's Not in Your Head, It's Your Hormones- Melinda Bonk
Cycles of Life-Ellen Kamhi
Natural Hormone Balance-Uzzi Reiss
Keep Your Breasts- Susan Moss
Breast Health- Charles Simone
How to Prevent Breast Cancer- Ross Pelton
Recovery From Cancer- Elaine Nussbaum
The Truth About Breast Cancer- Joseph Keon
Complete Idiots Guide to Fasting- Eve Adamson
The Okinawan Program- Bradley Willcox
The Miracle of Fasting- Patricia Bragg
Miracle Results of Fasting- Dave Williams
Recalled by Life- Anthony Satarillo
Macrobiotic Miracle- Virginia Brown
Healthy Eating for Life- PCRM
Live Longer, Live Better- Neal Barnard (anything by Neal)
Healthy Fasting- Norbert Kriegisch
Fast Your Way to Health- Lee Bueno
Fasting- and Eating- for Life- Joel Fuhrman
Fasting- The Ultimate Diet- Alan Cott
The 120 Year Diet, and Maxiumum Lifespan- Roy Walford

YOUR BASIC HORMONES

Androstenedione- the second major androgen

Cortisol- the stress hormone

DHEA- dehydroepiandrosterone

Estradiol- E2 the most powerful estrogen

Estriol- E3 the safe estrogen

Estrone-E1 the second strongest estrogen

FSH- follicle stimulating hormone

Growth Hormone- the pituitary hormone

LH- luteinizing hormone

Melatonin- secreted by the pineal gland

Pregnenolone- the brain hormone

Progesterone- the progestation hormone

Prolactin- for milk secretion

Testosterone- the major androgen

T3- triiodothyronine thyroid

T4- L-thyroxine thyroid

OTHER BOOKS AVAILABLE FROM SAFE GOODS

Eye Care Naturally	$ 8.95 US $12.95 CAN
Lower Cholesterol Without Drugs- Roger Mason	$ 6.95 US $10.95 CAN
The Natural Prostate Cure - Roger Mason	$ 6.95 US $10.95 CAN
Zen Macrobiotics for Americans- Roger Mason	$ 7.95 US $11.95 CAN
What Is Beta Glucan?- Roger Mason	$4.95 US $6.95 CAN
Natural Born Fatburners	$14.95 US $22.95 CAN
Cancer Disarmed Expanded	$ 6.95 US $10.95 CAN
Dr.Vagnini's Healthy Heart Plan	$16.95 US $24.95 CAN
Overcoming Senior Moments	$7.95 US $11.95 CAN

For a complete listing of books visit our web site:
www.safegoodspub.com
or call for a free catalog (888)628-8731
order line: (888) NATURE-1